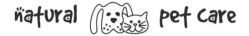

natural pet care

Arthritis

D0797101

BY LISA S. NEWMAN, N.D., Ph.D

Foreword by Deborah C. Mallu, D.V.M., C.V.A.

THE CROSSING PRESS
FREEDOM, CALIFORNIA

For information on bulk purchases or group discounts for this and other Crossing Press titles, please contact our Special Sales Manager at 800/777-1048. Visit our web site: **www.crossingpress.com**

Cautionary Note: The nutritional information, recipes, and instructions contained within this book are in no way intended as a substitute for medical counseling. Please do not attempt self-treatment of a medical problem without consulting a qualified health practitioner.

The author and The Crossing Press expressly disclaim any and all liability for any claims, damages, losses, judgments, expenses, costs, and liabilities of any kind or injuries resulting from any products offered in this book by participating companies and their employees or agents. Nor does the inclusion of any resource group or company listed within this book constitute an endorsement or guarantee of quality by the author or The Crossing Press.

Library of Congress Cataloging-in-Publication Data

Newman, Lisa S.
    Arthritis / by Lisa S. Newman.
        p. cm. -- (The Crossing Press pocket series)
    At head of title: Natural pet care.
    ISBN 1-58091-003-3 (pbk.)
    1. Dogs--Diseases--Alternative treatment. 2. Cats--Diseases-
-Alternative treatment. 3. Arthritis in animals. 4. Holistic
veterinary medicine. I. Title. II. Title: Natural pet care.
III. Series.
SF992.A77N48   1999
636.7'0896722--dc21
                                        99-37386
                                          CIP

Contents

Foreword

It is with great pleasure that I introduce Lisa Newman's remarkable series. She has dedicated her life to helping you care for your animal companions—we can all benefit from her years of experience.

We are living in a time of great change, especially in the realm of health care. As a practicing veterinarian for more than two decades, I have witnessed both myself and my clients begin to seek less invasive, more natural methods for healing our dogs and cats. Once we understood that all beings are interconnected on this planet, we became aware that our thoughts, emotions, and family dynamics played an important role in the health of our animal companions. We began to realize the importance of forming a team first with the members of our animal family, aided by other healing professionals including natural health counselors and animal communicators.

Over the years I have heard people say, "I didn't know you could use that natural remedy or treatment on animals." Feel confident that you can help your animal companions where the healing is best—in your loving home. Our animals nurture us by giving us unconditional love. In turn, we can nurture them with fresh, live food and supplements, so that they can live a long and healthy life. Lisa Newman will show you the way so that you can be empowered as a healer.

Deborah C. Mallu, D.V.M., C.V.A.

Arthritis as a Symptom

Inbreeding and excessive genetic manipulation has minimized our animals' natural curative abilities and has left our animals very susceptible to bone and joint disorders, increasing the occurrence of arthritis. Years of vaccinations, chemical baths, flea/tick potions, dips/sprays, medications, and most importantly, poor-quality ingredients, artificial colors, preservatives, and by-products found in most pet foods and treats influence the animal's resistance to degenerative diseases such as arthritis.

It is important to distinguish a true genetic disorder from a depressed immune system. Although the holistic method of treatment is very similar in both cases, by defining arthritis and understanding the relationship between genetic and lifestyle issues, you will be better prepared to address your own animal's individual needs and effectively improve their condition, regardless of the cause.

The diagnosis of arthritis has become too inclusive. Many conditions, muscular, nerve, or joint dysfunction, torn ligaments, calcification, old age, and poor autoimmune function, are often explained as arthritic disease. Some inflammatory reactions are true pathological processes that are triggered by the interaction of specific allergens, often food-related. These resulting arthritic symptoms are caused by a sensitivity.

Holistically, I see all "arthritic reactions" strictly as symptoms, rather than conditions. Even true arthritic disorders, whether genetically or environmentally triggered, are typically just a form of a hypersensitivity reaction. A specific arthritic reaction is a symptom: its underlying cause is rarely from the bones or joints themselves. Because it is difficult to distinguish between symptoms and causes, making a causative diagnosis and implementing a successful treatment protocol can be difficult.

Therapies focused only on the removal of the disorder (by surgery, for example) or suppression of the arthritic response, rather than addressing the root cause, will give symptomatic relief at best. At worst, they will cause chronic, more frequent cycling of the symptoms, which places enormous burdens on the body. This will happen even if the therapy you choose is a holistic one.

You must look beyond the symptoms or diagnosis. Certainly, I do not advocate allowing an animal to suffer in pain without addressing it. But, looking deeper, for the cause of the inflammation or pain, and addressing that imbalance will be more effective. It will reverse the symptom faster, and may prevent it from reoccurring.

In this chapter I will discuss the most commonly diagnosed arthritic disorders. You may be able to match your pet to one of the groups or you may have already received a similar diagnosis. If you explore more deeply, you may find that the underlying cause is not simply a structural or neurological problem. This deeper exploration may help you relieve or reverse your pet's symptoms.

DEFINING ARTHRITIS

There are three types of arthritis. The first type of condition is genetic. Pets who have chronic arthritis, and whose symptoms are more localized (hips, etc.) and predictable, are often diagnosed with genetically predisposed arthritis. Symptoms associated with genetically predisposed arthritis can include:

- poor structural development and stability
- bone loss and brittle condition

- over-calcification and stiff joints
- weak muscles and ligaments
- slow recovery from structural injury

Post-injury symptoms are most often referred to as arthritis. These symptoms are caused by the body's inability to return to a healthy state. The recurrence of symptoms related to a previous trauma, such as an accident that resulted in broken bones, a fight which caused joint dislocation, or even previous surgeries, can be almost impossible to eliminate completely. If an allopathic treatment of symptom suppression is adopted, animals seem to develop a tolerance to prescribed or over-the-counter anti-inflammatory drugs fairly quickly. Pain control often becomes less effective each year, leaving both owner and pet frustrated.

A holistic approach may prove more successful for animals who have either a genetic predisposition to arthritis or who have suffered traumatic injuries. By addressing the underlying immune system imbalance and stimulating the body's natural curative potential, an holistic protocol will quickly reverse chronic arthritic symptoms, and often completely eliminate the underlying weaknesses responsible.

While symptom suppression alone can be successfully accomplished through natural methods, a complete holistic protocol of detoxification, nutritional, and herbal supplementation is best. This approach will stimulate the immune system, and lead to a more rapid, and possibly thorough, reversal of arthritic symptoms.

The third type of arthritic symptoms are often associated with chemical or environmental irritants, particularly in aged pets. General arthritic symptoms can be exacerbated by environmental or chemical allergens, such as pollen or dips, or by weather changes. Arthritis can be triggered by specific foods and treats, and by by-products and chemicals

7

in foods, such as preservatives and artificial flavors. In addition to arthritis these pets can have low vitality, organ failure, and even exhibit excessive emotional/behavioral traits such as shyness, nervousness, or fear-aggression.

Arthritis is, in my opinion, the most misdiagnosed of conditions. There are over two hundred different commercial and prescription "senior" diets, yet our pets still suffer from fatigue, stiffness, pain, and restricted mobility. "Lite" or fiber-rich diets used to lighten the body's load on weak joints, have caused additional weight or bowel problems instead. This evidence points to other causes of arthritic symptoms. I believe the problem lies with the poor quality of the ingredients in our pet's food and the body's inability to digest and assimilate them.

Beef was one of the first ingredients targeted by veterinarians as a prime allergen associated with joint inflammation. Many pets, who previously tested positive for a beef sensitivity, are now eating high-quality beef regularly with no arthritic symptoms. Urea toxicity triggers inflammation.

Chemically irritated pets have a reaction to certain substances in their environment, including carpeting, shampoos, cigarette smoke, household cleaning products, vaccinations, pesticides, and even their own drinking water, beds, or collars. Chemical irritants can be produced by the body itself, for example, hormones. Or there may be insufficient chemical output from the endocrine system, as in the case of cortisol deficiency. Stress on other glands, such as the thyroid or pituitary, may also result from or contribute to arthritis. There is a wide range of symptoms associated with environmental irritants:

- reactive or infectious arthritis, especially rheumatism
- gastric upset including bloating, as chemicals interfere with digestion

- gas, diarrhea and/or constipation, irritable bowels
- vomiting, hair balls
- skin problems including dandruff, hot spots, pimples, redness, and itching
- poor coat condition including dry or greasy fur, coat loss, or fur picking
- ear and eye discharges and irritation
- general loss of vitality
- organ failure from chronic symptoms such as Feline Urological Syndrome (F.U.S.), cystitis, diabetes, and even poor elimination
- excessive emotional/behavioral traits such as complete isolation, nervousness, fearfulness, or aggression
- seizures
- cataracts
- diabetes
- cancer, especially fatty skin tumors, sarcomas, and leukemia
- loss of reproductive capabilities
- general immune dysfunction

This type of chemically based reactive arthritis is surprisingly common. Pets respond to their environment much as we do, reacting similarly to chemicals polluting their bodies. In some instances, our pets are exposed to far more chemicals than we ever are. Cats and dogs typically eat up to one-third their body weight in chemical preservatives each year, and are completely doused in chemical pesticides, which are then left on to be absorbed through the skin. When was the last time you took a bath in a lethal pesticide or wore a pesticide-laced collar daily? Or received yearly vaccinations?

Many pets spend much of their time in direct contact with carpeting, floors, and landscapes that have been heavily treated with cleaning solutions, herbicides, and pesticides. Repeated exposure makes them more likely to develop sensitivities to these chemicals. Pets may spend their day outside breathing car exhaust, and their night inside, exposed to second-hand smoke. Even drinking water may be a culprit if it contains heavy metals, chemicals, bacteria, and amoebas. If you are not willing to drink your own tap water, then please do not give it to your animals.

Many pets may also suffer from multiple conditions. The symptoms and resulting decline of health can be overwhelming. It is impossible to affect one part of the body without affecting the rest. Chronic drug use may result in organ failure. Death can occur, caused by the continual assault upon the body, especially the immune system. Too often, a pet is euthanized to end its suffering when even drugs can no longer suppress the symptoms.

I do not advocate allowing an animal to suffer unnecessarily. I recommend using a medication prescribed by your veterinarian in the event of a life-threatening imbalance, infection, or injury. However, I do strongly urge that we first change your pet's diet and improve its digestion and environment to strengthen its body. Drugs should be seen as a last resort, warranted only in an emergency, as in the case of anaphylactic shock, adrenal malfunction, or to ward off life-threatening paralysis. Consult with a veterinarian you trust, and weigh the pros and cons of various treatments.

Assessing Arthritis

To assess the nature of your pet's arthritic response and its severity, you must incorporate information that includes:

- how acute (immediate) or chronic (long-term) the onset of symptoms are
- the time (upon rising or after exercise) or weather in which it is most aggravated
- exposure to emotional and environmental stress, including poor diet
- clinical tests and x-rays

The allopathic veterinary practitioner will focus on the diagnosis of "arthritis" and will seek to suppress symptoms through drugs (antibiotics, pain relief, and steroids for inflammation). All too often, there is a full return of symptoms shortly after medication is terminated.

The holistic practitioner, on the other hand, will use these assessments as confirmation of an underlying imbalance. Initially, those ingredients, which have tested positive as an allergen and trigger inflammation, may be avoided, and certain symptoms suppressed (preferably naturally). Emphasis is placed on reversal of the condition through stimulation of the body's defense mechanisms (immune system) which may eliminate the symptoms altogether. In a large majority of animals, holistic animal care often allows the reintroduction of the very ingredients previously known to have triggered an arthritic response.

ARTHRITIS: GENETIC PREDISPOSITION OR TOXICITY?

Let us now explore and evaluate what arthritis truly is and determine how often genetic predisposition or toxicity are the true culprits behind the "arthritic" reaction. In my experience, there is an overemphasis by veterinarians and pet store owners on arthritic symptoms rather than on investigating why and how the body reacts as it does. Often, the animal's symptoms are cyclic, changing from diet to diet, or from one supplement to another, with medications used to suppress the resulting symptoms. With each cycle or cold weather season, the arthritic response becomes worse and more difficult to treat. Short-term relief is generally successful, as long as the body remains responsive to medication. Eventually, more serious symptoms and other progressive diseases can develop.

Clinical examination and x-rays can identify a genetic disorder or injury while blood tests may be able to determine the body's biochemical processes, but, unfortunately, tests and examinations do little to reveal a complete picture of the arthritic weakness. Often, detective work on the part of the owner will uncover the causes of the arthritic symptoms.

Blood work can reveal the presence of various markers, such as histamine, lymphocytes, and antibodies to specific allergens (i.e., beef or urea—a waste by-product of beef proteins). These markers indicate that the immune system has marshaled a defense in which bruising from internal or external trauma causes visible localized joint swelling and stiffness. They do not show us if that specific source is the actual allergen, or whether a toxic level of waste from that source is the allergen. For example, if beef protein is compromised (i.e., diseased tissue or non-digestible sources of protein such as hide or hooves), and the body had a difficult time digesting and assimilating it, then a higher quantity of waste product would circulate in the blood. These toxins could trigger a release of histamines (causing joint inflammation), but the blood work would only be able to reveal that beef is an allergen. A standard course of treatment would recommend the elimination of beef and beef by-products to treat the inflammatory condition. This same pet, supported holistically and presented with a higher-quality beef diet, will no longer exhibit symptoms.

This dilemma is at the crux of the arthritis treatment firestorm. In holistic circles, this process is known as a "sensitivity." For example, if your body is constantly processing filth, it will eventually begin to respond to the filth, which could cause the joints to become sensitive and irritated. Imagine that the body is submersed in a vat of filth ten hours per day, and the prescribed treatment for the resultant skin problems is a fifteen-minute shower and the application of medicated creams two or three times a day. How quickly do you think the skin would heal completely? Would it ever have a chance to heal completely, if it is exposed daily, for hours at a time, to the source of irritation?

The same scenario is true for filth inside the body. It remains in contact with the mucous membranes in the digestive tract (interfering with proper assimilation), irritating the nervous system (reducing natural pain control), weakening the immune system (undermining joint repair and strengthening), and imbalancing the glandular system (interfering with all biological processes). The eliminatory system becomes burdened and unable to filter (detoxify) this filth.

To the holistic practitioner, the causes of this cycle are understandable. Our pets are constantly bombarded with chemicals, by-products, vaccinations, etc., and subjected to life in a symbolic "vat" of filth. When a substance is not easily broken down, absorbed and eliminated by the body, a build-up of waste results. Toxic levels of waste stimulate the immune system to release agents to corral and eliminate the culprit (hence, the positive results in blood work-ups).

But, the condition cannot be reversed by repeated suppression of arthritic symptoms with chemical treatment. This cycle of symptom suppression sentences thousands of pets to a lifetime of pain and suffering and perpetuates the myth that arthritis cannot be cured.

The Underlying Imbalance

The diagnosis of "arthritis" has steadily increased over the past ten years, even though, in the 1980s, several valuable studies were published which identified important factors to aid in the understanding, prevention, and treatment of arthritic conditions. These studies revealed that free radicals, especially toxins from meat, animal fat, and grain metabolism of commercial pet food ingredients can undermine general health. These reports also emphasized the detrimental effects of improper breeding practices that result in genetically crippled animals and rampant disease. For the most part, this information has been ignored by veterinarians and breeders.

Pet food companies have manufactured new and improved diets for arthritic symptoms based on new sources of animal protein, rather than the traditional beef, meat meal and bone meal, pork by-products and "other" animal by-products. Unfortunately, these new sources, lamb, lamb meal and bone meal, poultry by-products, fish by-products, and "other" animal by-products, are not too different from the old.

The use of chemicals in pet foods has not declined significantly. Instead, there are more chemicals and by-products being fed to our pets today under the guise of a "natural" or "senior" product! The fundamental quality of the diet is still sadly lacking.

Breeders continue to breed animals known to have a predisposition towards structural disorders. Veterinarians continue to use prednisone, pain medication, and antibiotics, but misunderstand the true benefit in some of these arthritic cases. Adrenal deficiency is seen in many chronically symptomatic pets. Corticosteroids can promote cortisol production, which stimulates and strengthens the immune system and aids in the reversal of inflammation. There is simple blood work that can be used to determine which animals will profit from steroids (to reverse a deficiency), and which animals would benefit from hormone therapy instead of the shotgun approach commonly used on any pet with similar symptoms. This method of identification is very helpful for those pets with true deficiencies that should be treated chemically. For the other animals, the immune system would have an opportunity to be stimulated naturally through nutritional, herbal, and homeopathic supplementation, rather than burdened further by medications not truly needed.

The quality and freshness of the ingredients in food plays a major role in triggering an arthritic response. It is not necessarily the ingredient itself that promotes the condition. Certainly, one should always seek to eliminate a food ingredient that may be an allergen, but there should be a greater focus on the body's ability to properly digest and assimilate nutrition and eliminate waste. The repair and maintenance of healthy cells for a strong immune system is essential to the elimination of your pet's arthritis.

Even if medication is needed, your pet's lifestyle can be enriched through holistic animal care. You will succeed if you honor life as nature's gift to your animal and use a holistic style to fully stimulate your pet's natural healing abilities.

What Is Holistic Animal Care?

Rather than simply addressing an animal's symptoms, holistic animal care addresses the whole body: body, mind, spirit, and even the environment. Different health modalities are used in a synergistic way to help stimulate, strengthen, and support the body's own biological processes and natural defenses.

Nutrition, which can often be the deciding factor between health and disease, is central to holistic care. It doesn't matter what number of drugs or natural remedies are given to a pet, if the pet is not receiving adequate nutrition, it will be lacking the basic tools with which to support its own recovery.

Nutrition is also the cornerstone of a modality known as naturopathy. Defined by a medical dictionary as "a drugless system of therapy by the use of physical forces, such as air, light, water, heat, massage, etc.," naturopathy is a comprehensive approach that emphasizes supporting the body's physical attempts to eliminate disease. Naturopaths believe that a major cause of disease is an excessive build-up of toxic materials (often due to improper eating and lack of exercise) which clog the eliminatory system. Various techniques are used to clean out (detoxify) the body and stimulate the reversal of symptoms and chronic dis-ease. The cleansing process is supported with high-quality nutrition, proper food combining (to stimulate and aid digestion), nutritional supplements, and herbs.

Herbs have been widely used by every culture since ancient times to stimulate healing. It is widely believed that people began using herbs after observing wild animals who instinctively select appropriate herbs when they are ill. Herbalists use specific leaves, roots, bark, flowers, and seeds to assist the healing process, primarily by helping detoxify the body. Herbs provide a slower and deeper action than pharmaceutical drugs.

Another modality, which also provides a slower and deeper action, is homeopathy. Sometimes nutrition or herbs can begin the cleansing process and support the body so that it can go cure itself. But often it is the homeopathic remedy which can stimulate the deeper levels of healing. The homeopathic system is safe, its basic principles are elegantly simple, and homeopathic remedies have been exhaustively researched and used successfully for hundreds of years.

The German physician, Samuel Hahnemann, founded homeopathy in the late 1700s. The basic principle of homeopathy is "Like will cure like." This principle was recognized by ancient Chinese masters of the healing arts, Hindu sages, as well as our history's most noted physicians and alchemists, Hippocrates and Paracelsus. Hahnemann's "provings"—that a substance that can mimic symptoms helps cure the symptoms—revolutionized the understanding of symptoms and disease. Trained as a physician, Hahnemann treated symptoms as unhealthy responses of the body that should be suppressed. He later learned that symptoms can be positive, adaptive responses to stresses that the body experiences. Hahnemann recognized that symptoms represented the body's effort to heal itself, and therefore our aim should be to stimulate, rather than suppress, the body's natural defenses.

Hahnemann noted certain similarities between symptoms produced by some diseases and by the very drugs used to treat them. From this he formed his "Law of Similars," postulating that a disease could be cured by whatever medicine produces similar symptoms when given to a healthy person. The beauty of homeopathic treatment is that it cooperates, rather than competes, with the body's own efforts to regain health.

A simplified example of how homeopathy works is that of bee venom. We know that a bee sting will cause swelling, fluid accumulation, redness of the skin, pain and soreness that is accentuated by the application of heat or pressure. Sensitive animals will also experience mental (emotional) symptoms such as apathy, stupor, listlessness, or the opposite, whining and fearfulness. If a homeopathically prepared dilute solution of bee venom (known as Apis) is given to a pet with these symptoms—even if the symptoms are caused by arthritis rather than a bee sting—the condition will soon begin to clear up. The key is that the symptoms are quite similar to what the remedy, in its undiluted state, would create. Flower essences (which balance emotional states) and tissue cell salts (which support physiological processes) act similarly, by stimulating the body's own natural healing and homeostasis.

THE HOLISTIC PET

A healthy, holistically reared pet is in a state of balance that exists on three interrelated levels: the physical, the emotional, and the environmental. A healthy pet experiences physical vitality and is free from physiological malfunction, displays emotional clarity resulting in good behavior and happiness, and receives (as well as contributes) joy, love, and security in their living environment.

This animal is the opposite of a chemically reared pet, who is often found to be in a state of imbalance or dis-ease. This animal lacks physical vitality and suffers from chronic symptoms due to physiological malfunction, displays emotional stress resulting in negative behavior, and often also lives in a physically toxic environment. Since it is impossible to have one organ system affected without it affecting the other organ systems, a system that is not in balance is more susceptible to assault.

Holistic animal care is simple and safe to use. *Treat the body well and the body will be well.* By providing the body with sufficient amounts of high-quality food, correct supplements, and holistic modalities when appropriate, the body will remain in a state of balance. If the balanced body is assaulted by certain substances, which create an imbalance, it has the strength to trigger the curative process and reestablish its balance.

THE ARTHRITIC PET

Some pets who are born genetically compromised develop structural disorders, such as hip dysplasia. Most of the pets who were not born genetically compromised also suffer from arthritis because they are exposed to chemicals and an emotionally and/or physically toxic environment. Chemicals alter the body's primary biological functions, place undue stress on vital organs and glands necessary for proper immune function, and destroy healthy ligament, joint, and muscular tissue. Arthritic pets have often been exposed to:

- standard commercial pet foods
- artificial treats
- shotgun medications (the indiscriminate use of "standard" medications)
- excessive vaccinations and yearly boosters
- toxic cleaning and pest-control products (especially collars or monthly drug doses)
- environmental pollution (without the benefit of regular detoxification)
- an emotionally and/or physically stressful living environment (past and present)

Commercial Foods Increase
Susceptibility to Arthritis

Commercial pet diets and treats are the primary reason pets develop all types of inflammatory responses, including food allergies, which can cause arthritic symptoms. It should be noted that the quality of the ingredient can do more harm and is more likely to trigger a response than the ingredients themselves. The standard use of by-products and meat sources unfit for human consumption severely limits the pet's ability to digest and assimilate nutrients well. The use of artificial colors or flavors, chemical preservatives, nitrates, and rancid animal fats also interfere with digestion. Poorly digested matter becomes harder to eliminate, causing a backup of old fecal material in the bowel, which further prohibits assimilation of vital nutrients needed to reverse structural dysfunction.

We can call this the screen door effect. Here in the desert where I live, we love screen doors and the ventilation that they provide. But we also struggle with blowing dirt and, on the few days of the season when it rains, my screen door can become caked with dirt. If I go out and brush it off right away there is not much of a problem, but if I wait a day or two the dirt can harden, especially if it rains again. Rain adheres the top layers of dirt more firmly onto the previous ones and can create an adobe mud effect, where the dirt becomes so hard that it cannot be brushed away and actually begins to block the flow of air.

This is similar to what happens inside a poorly maintained colon. Imagine the colon as the screen door to the body and nutrients are the air. As improperly digested matter moves into the colon and complete evacuation is not encouraged (mostly pets lack exercise, and can't always go outside to have a bowel movement), old fecal material begins to "collect." This material lines the walls of the colon, and chemicals (such as ethoxyquin, a commonly used pet food preservative that prohibits moisture absorption) make the feces so dry they cannot move easily down the colon. Moreover, this drying affects the size and hardness of the stools.

Most pet food companies will tell you that these stools mean their food is more "digestible with less waste to pick up." What do you think a medical doctor would say to you, if you described your own stools as coming out like that? Certainly, a better-quality food will produce less stool volume (generally due to less fillers first, better digestibility second), but it should not be from lack of moisture in the stool.

As old fecal material builds up inside the colon, the "screen door effect" begins. It becomes harder and harder for the body to clean out this material on its own. This interferes with the body's ability to absorb (or "ventilate") nutrients from digested matter in the colon into the bloodstream, to use for distribution among the body's hungry cells and energy-depleted organ systems.

The harder the pet food ingredients are to break down and process, and the more chemicals that are present, the more stress is placed on the body's functions. The harder the body has to work, the quicker it breaks down and falls apart. With improper digestion and assimilation, the body cannot utilize nutrients that are vital to proper biological processes such as immunity (resistance to degenerative processes). Improper digestion and assimilation also leads to a build-up of general waste (toxins) in the body, which places a huge burden upon the eliminatory organs. As the liver and kidneys become burdened, the body attempts to detoxify through the largest eliminatory organ it has, the skin, which leads to the development of skin and coat problems normally associated with allergies and is often seen in pets who develop arthritis. Additionally, the lymphatic and endocrine systems are overstimulated, possibly leading to the development of a deeper, more serious disease like cancer.

Chemicals in Non-Foods

A pet may also be exposed to chemicals and irritants in other, non-dietary, forms. Whether the irritant is a chemical-based breath mint given as a treat, an annual vaccination booster, an artificially perfumed shampoo, a medicated skin treatment, flea or tick control products, household cleaning agents, or long-term medication, any or all can have a detrimental effect on your animal's health. If you think of the healthy body as a balanced scale, when you continually add these chemicals to one side of the scale, it will remain out of balance, but if you add good nutrition and minimize the build-up of chemicals on the other, this scale stays in balance, preventing or reversing the arthritic process.

Other Factors Creating Imbalance in a Pet

It is important to recognize and address other factors that may cause imbalance and interfere with homeostasis. Structural imbalances are often a prime cause of dis-ease. Old injuries or genetic malfunctions, such as rheumatoid arthritis, can place stress on certain organ systems. A build-up of calcium deposits and joint or spinal inflammation may also put pressure on nerves involved with digestive organs, such as the stomach. This pressure can interfere with the normal function of the stomach and lead to improper digestion and assimilation of nutrients. Often, addressing the structural problems will help to reverse other disease as well. Chiropractic adjustments, massage, acupressure, and acupuncture can all be beneficial tools in your fight against your animal's poor condition.

Another issue that can cause imbalance is a stressful environment. Have you ever felt "a pain in the neck" and experienced muscular spasms due to a stressful situation? Pets who often experience extreme emotions (fear, nervousness, and tension) are also more likely to suffer from digestive problems and glandular imbalances, which may exacerbate arthritic symptoms. Sources of environmental stress include family changes such as relocating, members leaving or dying, divorce or new births, new jobs, etc. The pituitary, adrenal, and thyroid glands may be injured by chronic emotional stress. These glands are associated with the "fight or flight" reaction to negative stimuli. A safe and nurturing environment will ensure your pet's emotional well-being. The use of nutritional supplementation and remedies, especially flower essences, to re-balance the emotions can often be the key to a more complete physical healing.

When an animal is out of balance, waste builds up not only in the colon but also in the bloodstream, joints, and eliminatory organs. Urea, a waste product of meat protein metabolism, can cause arthritic conditions and also accounts for the high number of pets who test positive for meat allergies. The poorer the quality of meat and the more difficult it is to digest, the more waste is produced during digestion. Urea toxicity manifests itself in certain notable symptoms:

- premature aging with chronic arthritic symptoms
- known or suspected allergies to beef, pork, meat, meat by-products, or meat meal
- excessive licking and chewing of paws, resulting in edema and lick granuloma
- prickly heat-type rashes, itchy skin, with or without small pimples or pustules

- excessive loss of hair or coat condition
- foul-smelling breath, flatulence, and/or stool
- increased fatty tumor, cyst, or cancerous tumor production
- liver, pancreatic, gall bladder, and kidney dysfunction
- weakened immune responses, especially chronic skin infections
- parasitic infestation, especially fleas and ticks (which feed off skin-eliminated waste)
- neurological issues, including seizures
- aggression and other behavioral problems

Yeast, another nasty ingredient, is found in the majority of commercial pet diets, treats, supplements, flea and tick control products, and even many pet medications. Yeast, which is noted for its anti-flea and tick properties, is in practically everything! A cheap filler ingredient, it does provide some B vitamins, minerals, amino acids, and natural flavor to products, but is mostly used to increase the food's volume.

The most common form of yeast found in animal products is brewer's yeast, which is a waste product that has most of its nutrients eliminated during the brewing process. Yeast was long touted as a good source of nutrients, but we are now finding that this is not so. Nutritional yeast, a cultivated product, is nutritionally superior to brewer's yeast and tastier, but it still is not the best source of nutrients and, like brewer's yeast, it can be difficult to digest. Adequate levels of B vitamins are only available through supplements. It would take far too much yeast to provide an equivalent amount. Moreover, excessive yeast clogs the liver and increases general toxicity. According to recent veterinary research, arthritic animals are more likely to be allergic to yeast than to most other food sources. Yeast triggers joint inflammation.

Humans, too, do not digest yeast well. Poor digestion places an additional burden on the liver, resulting in inflammatory conditions. Chinese medicine recognizes the correlation between the liver and inflammation. Yeast supplementation, often prescribed by vets and alternative practitioners, is the culprit. Yeast may initially improve pets' mobility, but then the pet's arthritis often becomes more intense and more difficult to treat, which can cause liver toxicity symptoms, including joint inflammation. I always recommend detoxification and the total elimination of yeast and sugar (which compounds yeast toxicity) from animals' diets for six weeks. Other than a daily multiple vitamin/mineral supplement (high in B vitamins and Vitamin C) and a natural anti-inflammatory, nothing else was used to treat their arthritic condition, yet it would quickly resolve on its own.

One of my human clients who had suffered from a degenerative joint disease for years and had been diagnosed as having chronic liver problems, tested positive for a yeast allergy. Three months later, under my guidance, he was given a clean bill of health and had a negative reaction for a yeast allergy! We then reintroduced yeast into his diet and he never had another arthritic flare-up, as long as he did not deviate from his holistic lifestyle.

Yeast toxicity manifests itself in certain symptoms, most notably:

- premature aging with arthritic manifestation and possibly digestive symptoms
- known or suspected allergies to yeast or yeast-containing foods such as dry kibble
- ear infections, eye discharges, and upper respiratory problems, including asthma
- excessive licking and chewing of the body and face rubbing
- hot spots, itchy skin, with or without small pimples or pustules
- slower healing of tissue, including ligaments
- excessive loss of fur or coat condition

- foul-smelling breath, flatulence, and/or stool (especially off-colored stool with mucus)
- increased fatty tumor, cyst, or cancerous tumor production
- poor digestion and assimilation of other nutrients
- blood sugar instability
- high levels of liver enzymes and eosinophils (represents a damaged liver)
- liver, spleen, gall bladder, and/or pancreatic dysfunction including diabetes
- weakened immune responses, especially chronic infections
- increased sensitivities to pollution, vaccinations, and chemicals in general
- aggression, fearful-aggressive, or fearful behavior in certain pets
- parasitic infestation, especially fleas and ticks (who feed off skin-eliminated waste)

As urea, metabolized yeast, and other excess waste builds up in the body, undue stress is placed upon vital organs. First, the ability to break down nutrients is reduced, waste begins to circulate, and fewer nutrients are available to stimulate the body's defenses. Next the eliminatory, lymphatic, and immune systems become burdened. Chronic symptoms develop—notably those diagnosed as "arthritis"—and suppression of the symptoms is initiated. Once medication is stopped, the symptoms return and the cycle continues. Ultimately, there is organ and gland malfunction, possibly leading to an early death.

Any pet suffering from structural disorders, sensitivities, old age, or injury (all of which may result in arthritis) can benefit from holistic animal care. Regardless of the symptoms, the underlying causes are fundamentally the same. A wholesome, toxin-free approach to diet and environment can not only prevent an arthritic symptom, but can also reverse it more quickly and effectively than the further application of chemicals.

Holistic Reversal of Arthritis

To reverse the underlying weakness that can manifest as arthritic symptoms, a holistic animal care lifestyle should be followed or there is a risk that symptoms will only be suppressed temporarily. Whether your pet's condition is a genetic disorder, injury, or reactive symptom, fasting and detoxification is an important first step. These processes help prepare the body for further re-balancing, and ultimately for healing. Changing to a natural, high-quality diet, supplemented with nutritional, herbal, and homeopathic products, provides the necessary foundation to stimulate the pet's natural healing ability.

Treating arthritis without first addressing a possible underlying nutritional imbalance is a waste of time. Diet may be a causative factor. Many treats, and even so-called "natural" supplements, are full of fillers such as yeast, chemicals, artificial flavors and colors. Look carefully at what you are feeding your pet. Re-balance a home-cooked diet, or find a better-quality commercial diet, and your pet's arthritis may be reversed.

To introduce a dietary change and initiate a successful arthritis relief program, begin by imposing a short twenty-four hour period of fasting. Many people associate fasting with deliberately starving their pet. Yet this couldn't be farther from the truth. Fasting can save your pet's life!

Fasting encourages the body to detoxify and re-balance. Old fecal material is expelled from the colon. Vital eliminatory organs—the kidneys and liver—are given a respite from processing waste, thus allowing a deeper processing of backed-up toxins to take place. Digestion and elimination, necessary processes for the uptake of nutrients and therapeutic substances such as anti-inflammatory herbs, are improved. The immune system, which helps the body resist arthritic responses, is strengthened and the overall condition of your pet is improved.

The fasting methods we will explore are very safe and gentle. People are bothered most when their pets look at them pleadingly at dinnertime. It is true that twenty-five percent of that pleading look may be caused by hunger, but you should know that the other seventy-five percent is definitely an attempt to control you. Pets, particularly dogs, are experts at controlling their masters. To avoid the pleading look during fasting, do something with your pet at their usual dinnertime that is fun. Bring home a new kitty toy (but, please not out of guilt!), or take your canine friend out for a fifteen-minute walk. These activities will not only occupy you and your pet's minds, but will also provide you both with much-needed exercise. If your pet cannot be fasted because of its physical condition, homeopathic detoxification works well by itself.

In order to encourage elimination still further during the twenty-four hour period of fasting, you can add a homeopathic remedy. This combination of fasting along with a homeopathic remedy is the fastest detoxification method. If you use the homeopathic remedy or the fasting alone, the process will take longer.

Anyone who has tried to clean with a dirty sponge can relate to the fact that once the sponge has been rinsed out, it becomes more effective at doing its job. Even a short twenty-four hour fast with homeopathic support can make a world of difference. Detoxification makes for better digestion and better assimilation of the vital nutrients necessary to help stimulate healing and strengthening. Without proper detoxification, the body's ability to cure itself is limited.

Once the detoxification process has occurred, usually within the first six to eight weeks, you will see a reversal of symptoms. In over seventy-five percent of cases I have observed, this method of detoxification, along with dietary changes and basic nutritional support, effectively reversed the "arthritic" condition.

In the remaining twenty-five percent of cases, including those with true joint disorder, arthritic degeneration, or other chronic debilitating dis-ease, the judicious use of homeopathic, herbal, and nutritional supplementation in a continuing course of treatment will definitely strengthen the animal's constitution and reduce, or eventually eliminate, their condition. With these cases, it can often take a couple of years for the body to eliminate the arthritis completely.

Treating your pet's arthritis holistically, rather than relying on symptom suppression, is the quickest, most effective way to reverse an arthritic (or any underlying) condition completely. With a systematic detoxification and strengthening program, the underlying condition will progressively improve, but the improvement may be subtle. Don't stop detoxification and supplementation as soon as symptoms have been suppressed because the body can become burdened again since it has a predisposition to this weakness, and will again respond to toxins or stress.

For pets with chronic dis-ease, the results of an ongoing holistic animal care program can be miraculous. As each year passes, the body will become stronger and less sensitive to toxins. With each arthritic episode, the animal will exhibit less severe symptoms, they become easier to treat, and there will be faster resolution. In those animals that are genetically or environmentally predisposed to deeper dis-ease, holistic animal care will minimize the possibility of degenerative conditions and maximize healing potential. At the very least, you will slow down the degenerative process.

Before starting a fasting program, check with your veterinarian. Perhaps your pet has diabetes and must maintain their blood sugar with food as well as insulin. Perhaps your veterinarian feels that your pet is too weak to fast, or your pet has had a recent bout of minor infections. It is always wise to rely on a trusted medical opinion, especially if you have a veterinarian who supports your holistic lifestyle.

There are two methods of fasting I recommend. The major difference to consider when deciding which fasting method is best for your pet is your pet's condition prior to starting the fast.

THE STANDARD FAST

The standard method is used for pets with acute or chronic arthritis that are otherwise in good health, and can adhere to a straight fast. Age makes no difference, as I have seen fasting succeed with a struggling one-week-old kitten or a 14-year-old dog.

Day One—Fast

Feed your pet breakfast as you normally would on the morning you are to begin the fast. Eliminate the evening meal. Be sure to provide plenty of fresh pure drinking water. Provide fun-filled activity in fresh air and sunshine, twice during the first day, followed by a damp terry cloth rubdown. Be sure not to overtire or place undue stress on your pet.

Day Two—Breaking the Fast

The following morning (after twenty-four hours of fasting) feed your pet one-half its usual breakfast. To make this process really special, break the fast with cooked oatmeal. It will absorb impurities in the digestive tract. To the oatmeal, you can add a teaspoon or two of raw honey, encapsulated garlic oil (raw garlic can be too harsh at this point), and some type of fresh green extract such as barley grass or spirulina. A fresh green extract can be very soothing and cleansing to the digestive system after fasting. Cats may prefer a little tuna water for flavor. Supplements can also be reintroduced into the diet at this time.

Provide exercise in the fresh air and sunshine twice on this second day, followed by a damp terry cloth rubdown. Remember plenty of water and be sure not to overtire or stress out your pet. For dinner, feed the normal quantity (and, hopefully, better quality) of food.

This is also a good fasting protocol to follow on a weekly basis to help maintain general health and well-being. Regarding this weekly fast, you will quickly find what suits you and your animal's own needs. Remember that exercise is very important at all times, but is especially important during cleansing to help move toxins out of the body by stimulating the eliminatory organs. The terry cloth rubdown also helps to stimulate the skin as it continues to process waste from the body's detoxification. If an odor is present during fasting, mix one-quarter cup of baking soda to one gallon of warm, purified water, rinse off the pet's body with this solution, and then dry it with a towel. The baking soda will help to neutralize the odor and balance the skin's pH, reducing any itching. Avoid using tap water, as it contains chlorine (a known skin irritant that will increase itching), which will be reabsorbed into the skin. If tap water is the only available water, boil it for fifteen minutes to help evaporate the chlorine. Be sure to let it cool down before using. A cut-up lemon boiled in the water for twenty minutes, then strained, acts as an additional deodorizer and disinfectant.

Generally, a standard twenty-four-hour fast is sufficient, but you may choose to follow it for two to three days longer if your pet was suddenly overcome by symptoms, is fighting an infection, has been on very poor-quality diets, or has not been eating well.

EXTENDED STANDARD FAST
Day One
Use the same protocol as the standard fast.

Day Two (and Possibly Day Three, Day Four)
Provide fun-filled activity in fresh air and sunshine twice during this day of fasting, followed by a damp terry cloth rubdown. Be especially sure not to overtire or place undue stress on your pet. Apple juice or vegetable juices (carrot, celery, or parsnip is best—avoid tomato juice) may be given in small amounts during the day, approximately one-quarter cup per twenty-five pounds of body weight per day. Do not over-do! These juices can also be frozen into small ice cubes for your pet's enjoyment during warmer months.

Breaking Fast Day
Break this fast with one-quarter of your pet's normal quantity of food in the morning, and the same (one-quarter) quantity for dinner. Both meals should be the cooked oatmeal. A little fruit or vegetable fiber (from juicing) can be also added to the oatmeal and future meals.

Second Day of Breaking Fast
Feed one-half normal rations in the morning and evening of the second day. Mix your pet's new natural diet fifty-fifty with cooked oatmeal.

Third Day of Breaking Fast

Feed full rations of a natural diet of your choice at breakfast and dinner. This is a good time to introduce fresh fruits and vegetables to your pet's diet on a regular basis.

THE ALTERNATIVE FASTING METHOD

An alternative fasting method may be more appropriate for pets with arthritis who also struggle with other serious conditions, such as cancer or diabetes, or are initially very debilitated and require additional nutritional and/or herbal support. To avoid huge dips in blood sugar and additional stress on the animal's biochemical balance, fasting should be limited to twenty-four hours. Actually, it is easier and almost as beneficial for the body to complete several twenty-four-hour fasts within a few weeks, even if there are only a few days break between each twenty-four-hour fast, rather than fasting for three or four consecutive days.

Day One

Feed your pet its usual breakfast. For the evening meal substitute a vegetable broth. To make this broth, grate equal amounts of fresh, raw carrots, beets, parsley, parsnips, spinach, and kale to a total of one cup of combined vegetables. Add grated vegetables to four cups of boiling water (avoid tap water) and simmer on low until all the vegetables are very soft, about twenty to thirty minutes. Separate the cooked vegetables and refrigerate to be used later. Refrigerate the broth in a well-sealed container.

Feed your pet one-half cup of broth per twenty pounds of body weight, per meal. You may give one or two additional meals of this broth during the fasting, if your animal seems to be very hungry, but do not overfeed in one sitting. Prior to feeding, warm the broth—but never in the microwave, which will destroy available nutrients. Cold broth may upset sensitive stomachs and lacks palatability. Prior to feeding the broth, give your pet orally any supplements or medications prescribed to be given with food.

Break Alternative Fast Day

The next morning feed your pet one-half the amount of broth you used during the preceding day, adding one-quarter the normal ration of food. Cooked oatmeal may be a good alternative to regular food during this fast breaking period, especially if there is a lot of colon cleansing needed. Repeat morning menu for the evening meal.

Second Day of Breaking the Alternative Fast

Feed one-half the amount of broth you used during the fast and add one-quarter the normal ration of food or one-eighth ration of food and one-eighth ration of cooked oatmeal. For the evening meal feed three-quarters the normal ration of food (no broth).

Third Day of Breaking the Alternate Fast

Introduce the full ration of your pet's natural diet at each meal.

This protocol will allow the body to begin detoxification without excess stress. When in doubt as to which process should be followed, it might be best to use the alternative fasting protocol. In a pinch, try cutting back twenty-five to fifty percent of their standard meal with the addition of nutritional supplements, herbal extracts, vegetable and fruit juices—which will also serve to stimulate a deeper elimination, without upsetting their metabolism.

SUPPORTIVE PHYTOCHEMICALS

The best detoxifying herbs, vegetables, and fruits (gentle enough to use now) are:

- *Milk Thistle* is good for liver cleansing and support, and helps process urea.
- *Dandelion* is an effective blood purifier and general organ cleanser.
- *Burdock Root* helps remove catabolic waste from cellular activity.
- *Slippery Elm* is very soothing to inflamed colon tissues and helps settle the stomach.
- *Yucca* is a natural anti-inflammatory, supports circulation, and reduces discomfort. Promotes kidney and liver detoxification.
- *Garlic* is anti-bacterial, anti-viral, anti-fungal, and anti-parasitic.
- *Kombu* is a sea vegetable that alkalizes the body and purifies the blood of fats.
- *Spirulina* is high in chlorophyll and aids enzyme production and digestion.
- *Carrots* are trace mineral-rich, high in vitamins, and alkalize the body.
- *Beets* provide several supportive nutrients, fiber, and flavor.
- *Parsnips* provide wonderful support for detoxifying the kidneys.
- *Spinach* is an excellent source of nutrients, especially trace minerals.
- *Celery* is trace mineral-rich, high in vitamins, alkalizing, and flavorful to pets.
- *Parsley* is trace mineral-rich, oxygenating to the blood, and helps detoxify odors.
- *Ginger* can help the digestive system, reduces gas, and aids in lowering hypertension.
- *Apples* provide needed energy while supporting detoxification.
- *Cranberries* are very high in Vitamin C, and help flush urinary tract waste.
- *Papaya* re-balances and aids digestion, and helps flush wastes.

Avoid highly acidic vegetables like tomatoes and onions (which can be deadly to dogs), or difficult-to-digest ingredients like cabbage. Also avoid using harsh fibers, such as psyllium, by themselves, as they can further irritate and damage sensitive intestinal tissues. Although a good ingredient for producing bulk and encouraging elimination, psyllium's negative side effects outweigh its benefits during detoxification.

HOMEOPATHIC DETOXIFICATION

Homeopathic detoxification encourages elimination and works well when combined with fasting, or used alone. One or several individual homeopathic remedies may be chosen, based on your pets' individual needs, or you may find that one of the many combination remedies available will work just as well. For detoxification and general symptom reversal it is best to work within the lower potencies, Xs to low Cs. Homeopathic detoxification should be used daily for no less than two weeks, preferably six to eight weeks. Give one daily dose at bedtime for most cases, or one dose upon rising and again at bedtime for more chronic cases.

Sometimes it is advisable to allow an initial build-up of the remedy by frequent dosing. Give one dose every fifteen minutes for the first hour (four times) when beginning detoxification and any other time you feel that your pet might need a little extra detoxifying boost. You cannot overdose your pet. Each repeated dose enhances the effect.

After the initial detoxification process, a maintenance program can be initiated on a weekly basis: a single weekly dose at bedtime to help process current waste build-up, stimulate proper kidney and liver function, and support general good health. It does not mean that homeopathic detoxification should be used in lieu of proper feeding, supplementation, and care. It should be used only as a support to biological functions such as digestion and elimination.

Homeopathic Remedies for Detoxification

- *Antimonium Crudum* is good for gout-like symptoms with gastric weaknesses.
- *Arsenicum Album* is used for general detoxification, re-balances the liver and spleen, and reverses the inflammatory response due to toxic joints.
- *Berberis Vulgaris* is good for a gouty constitution, particularly for a pet with a history of poor nutrition that is related to the onset of arthritis.
- *Bryonia* helps digestive problems contributing to waste build-up.
- *Cadium Sulph.* balances basic disease with gastric involvement.
- *Carduus Marianus* supports the vascular system, gall bladder, and liver.
- *Chelidonium Majus* is a liver remedy used for degenerative diseases.
- *Hydrastis* improves liver action and stimulates the immune system.
- *Juniperus Communis* encourages urine production and kidney elimination.
- *Solidago Vira* supports detoxification by eliminating free radicals through the kidneys.
- *Taraxacum* is used for bilious attacks and flatulence associated with cleansing.
- *Nux Vomica* helps to counter nausea, irritability, digestive disturbances, and portal congestion sometimes associated with the detoxification process.

Nux Vomica is often the first remedy homeopaths choose to establish equilibrium of biological functions and to counteract many chronic effects. It should always be included, regardless of what other remedies are chosen. The best homeopathic combinations for detoxification on the market today include this remedy. I have used *Arsenicum Album* and *Nux Vomica* to reverse many acute toxic reactions (including pesticide poisonings). When in doubt, this is a sound combination to try.

WHAT TO EXPECT
DURING DETOXIFICATION

Since detoxification removes waste from the body, waste will present itself during the detoxification process. Sometimes the very symptoms you are trying to address with the cleansing process are aggravated. This is a good sign! Called a curative response, it is a clear indicator that the body has been stimulated into cleansing. Curative responses are a natural part of detoxification and are vital to strengthening and re-balancing the body. When this response occurs, the first impulse many people have is to run to the veterinarian to get a drug to suppress the resulting symptoms. Don't do it!

In striving to reach your pet's fullest curative potential, it is vital to the process that symptoms be *supported* rather than *suppressed*. More so than at any other time, suppression of these symptoms—even through the use of holistic animal care, rather than drugs—will only force the underlying imbalance even deeper. The use of chemicals and medications at this time—especially steroids and antibiotics—will also severely burden the body and the cleansing process.

Sometimes people will prematurely terminate the cleansing process because they fear the return or worsening of their pet's symptoms. Although symptoms may have been suppressed only through natural methods, if the cleansing process is terminated prematurely, you and your pet will eventually have to go through the detoxification again if you can ever hope for true healing. It is best to address the symptoms gently (naturally), while continuing detoxification. Many things can be done to help minimize the aggravation (curative response) your pet experiences, without suppressing the cleansing and strengthening process. The safest, most effective way to support symptom aggravations is through the gentle modalities of nutritional supplements, homeopathy, flower essences, and herbs.

Please note that aggravations do not have to occur for a successful detoxification. It is more common for the process to happen relatively easily, regardless of the pet's previous condition.

Pets who seemed to be healthy prior to detoxification can exhibit the worst symptoms, perhaps from an imbalance that was suppressed long ago. The bottom line is that you must be aware of your own pet's individual process and support that, regardless of any preconceived notions you may have had regarding what the process should be like. Each time the body experiences a curative response, which has been supported rather than suppressed, the body is strengthened, and the symptoms will return less frequently and less aggressively until eventually the symptoms are eliminated (reversed) completely.

Please, do not forget the power of love. Spend time nurturing your pet even if only to respect their need to be quiet and sleep more during this process of symptom reversal. Such tenderness will certainly help minimize any stress they may be experiencing.

HINTS TO AID THE GENERAL DETOXIFICATION PROCESS

Provide plenty of pure water. Water is needed to help flush wastes as they are being eliminated. Avoid using tap water containing chlorine and chemicals (which may be too harsh for the kidneys to handle), or distilled water which may facilitate too rapid a detoxification. Be sure that your pet's drinking water is always free of metals and sediments.

Groom daily. Grooming is necessary to brush away toxins that are being eliminated though the skin. This also stimulates circulation, further aiding elimination. Removal of old, dead skin also stimulates the growth of new, healthier coats. Wipe away any ear, eye, penile, vaginal, or anal discharges to avoid infections.

Provide daily exercise in fresh air and sunshine. This is necessary to encourage respiration, which supports the removal of deeper toxins. This also improves your pet's attitude, which supports healing. For indoor-only cats or small dogs, please provide a screened-in area where fresh air and sunshine can still be enjoyed.

Respect your pet's quiet times. Do so even if the pet's withdrawal from interaction with the family troubles you. It is normal for pets going through detoxification to sleep more, continue the fasting process on their own when they need to, become irritable, or seek out warmer or cooler areas. When in doubt, do consult your veterinarian.

Avoid the use of all chemicals and drugs that are not absolutely necessary for sustaining life. They will severely interfere with the detoxification process and may even be more harmful to your pet during this time. As the cleansing process moves deeper into the body and joints, your pet's reaction to these substances may be stronger than usual, and it is possible there may be an allergic reaction!

Avoid giving a vaccine booster within six weeks prior to, or after, a deep detoxification. The body may have a harder time detoxifying shortly after a vaccination, or may react even more strongly than usual.

Address symptom aggravations gently through the use of nutritional supplementation, homeopathy, flower essences, or herbs. This will allow the cleansing process to continue while keeping the symptoms from becoming too uncomfortable for your pet.

Keep track of your pet's progress to help you better understand the process they are going through. If you jot down a few notes each day, you will be less likely to scare yourself into thinking that it has been days since your pet last ate, when it isn't true.

On the one hand, if three days ago your pet began displaying difficulty getting off the floor but was able to walk out of it and now cannot, you will need to add a natural anti-inflammatory such as yucca or SOD to reverse any possible toxicity that may have triggered the reaction. Then you will want to keep track of how many days stiffness and pain continues to be an issue, or how quickly your pet responded to the yucca, etc., so that you may seek out other support if needed. On the other hand, if you noted that the stiffness took two weeks to relieve—then returned in three weeks, but only took four days to reverse that time and did not return for two months the next time—then you begin to see a pattern that indicates you are on the right track!

COMMON SYMPTOMS OF DETOXIFICATION

Abscesses can erupt during the detoxification process, especially around the chest and back. As one of its defenses against toxins, the body will pocket an irritating substance or allergen (sometimes for years) to keep it from establishing a deeper hold on the body. Detoxification releases these toxins from the fatty tissue where they are stored and moves them back into the bloodstream for elimination. Since the skin is the largest eliminatory organ, abscesses may commonly occur. Abscesses also occur internally in the pockets surrounding the joints, eventually breaking the skin. At the first sign of swelling and accompanying heat, a dose of homeopathic *Belladonna* or *Sulphur* may discourage the full formation of an abscess.

Whether you suspect a foreign object or not, use the homeopathic remedy *Silica*, which encourages eruption and drainage. Since the abscess itself is actually a foreign object, *Silica* will generally work well. If not, try *Mercurius*, especially if thick pus has formed and the skin surrounding it has become angrier. Apply a warm, damp cloth to the area for fifteen minutes at a time to encourage eruption of the abscess, which will also soothe your pet. Homeopathic *Hepar Sulphuricum* is the best remedy for abscesses too painful to touch. *Apis* is excellent for abscesses that are located over joints and contribute to joint pain. Both can be used in conjunction with *Silica*.

Once there is drainage, be sure to keep the area clean and dry. It is helpful to trim away a little fur around the site to expose it to more air. This encourages healing, and makes it easier to treat the abscess topically. Clean it with a solution of fifty percent hydrogen peroxide and fifty percent water, then apply a little diluted *Tea Tree* or *Calendula* lotion to help encourage healing and prevent more severe infections. Treat topically at least once a day, twice a day if the abscess is large and angry. (See *Infections* in this chapter.)

Dehydration can occur when there is excessive vomiting or diarrhea, which causes an imbalance of nutrients and electrolytes. Dehydration will quickly shut down bodily functions, especially detoxification. To check for dehydration in a cat or small dog, grab the skin from the back of the neck between your forefinger and thumb, pull it gently upwards, and release it. In medium- to large-sized dogs, you can also press the side of the lip up and release it. The skin in either case should snap back into place within a second or two. If it takes longer, then dehydration is a problem. If you are concerned, consult your veterinarian immediately for subcutaneous fluid replacement therapy. In all other instances you can easily rehydrate your pet by encouraging them to drink water or by using a syringe, without a needle.

A pet should receive one ounce of water per pound of body weight, per day. Electrolyte solutions can be added to the water if the animal seems weakened by the dehydration. Ice cubes and water mixed into meals can also help.

Diarrhea can sometimes occur, especially as old fecal materials are processed, or as a side effect of general detoxification. One or two doses daily of homeopathic *Arsenicum* and *Nux Vomica*, helpful when nausea is also present, will generally firm up the stool while continuing to support elimination. If the diarrhea is severe or very watery, use this remedy more frequently, every fifteen minutes for the first hour and then every hour afterward, until the diarrhea is resolved. *Slippery Elm* is a soothing herb for the colon during and after a bout with diarrhea. In this case, use powdered *Slippery Elm* instead of the extract or tincture. To be certain that your animal is not dehydrating due to the loss of fluids through the diarrhea, watch how much water your pet drinks and check for the physical signs.

Discharges from all orifices are normal during detoxification. These are the routes that toxins can take directly out of the body. If your pet has a history of ear or eye irritations, nasal discharges, impacted anal glands (blocked discharge), mucous-coated stools, etc., you can expect an aggravation of these symptoms. Keep these areas clean, and utilize homeopathic remedies. *Arsenicum* is helpful as a general remedy, or you may want to explore others more directly suited to your pet's symptoms. Regardless of where these discharges originate, *Calcarea Carbonica* is an excellent constitutional remedy for watery to thicker discharges, and *Pulsatilla* is suited for discharges that are thick and yellow to greenish in color.

Dry, flaky skin can be easily cared for with a good brushing, terry cloth rubdown, and the application of some *Jojoba* or *Tea Tree* oil conditioner. Flaking of old skin cells is a normal part of detoxification, as old tissue is being replaced by healthier skin. One or two doses of homeopathic *Sulphur* can also be very beneficial at this time. *M.S.M.* is a nutritional sulfur supplement that helps tissue repair and growth. The herb *Horsetail* also contains a high concentration of naturally occurring sulfur.

Frequent bathing can rob the skin of necessary oils, causing an excessive release of these oils, which are the body's attempt to rebalance the skin. Avoid bathing your pet more than every few weeks.

Fever can be a good sign during detoxification, as long as the overall condition of the animal is stable. If you observe that your pet is severely exhausted, you may need to call a veterinarian. Fever supports detoxification, indicating that the body's defenses are working to burn up toxins and old viral or bacterial infections. If you suspect a fever after twenty-four hours of fasting or a few weeks of ongoing detoxification and dietary improvements, realize that this can be a normal part of the detoxification process. However, support is needed to keep the fever from weakening the body. Homeopathic remedies work best in this case. I highly recommend *Phosphorus*. If this fever is the result of an infection, increase garlic supplements, and add herbal products such as *Standardized Grapefruit Extract*, *Echinacea*, or *Golden Seal Root*, all excellent, safe natural antibiotics. If the fever is high, especially with debilitating side effects, or lasts more than two days, seek veterinary advice.

Flatulence can be a problem during cleansing, because old fecal material is being eliminated. Detoxification increases peristalsis (the muscular contractions of the colon,

which move fecal matter along and help to break it down).
It is like turning over a well-decomposed compost heap so
that the decayed material can be exposed and the odors
released into the air. A good dose of *Arsenicum* and *Nux
Vomica* will also help relieve flatulence.

Infections respond well to herbal support. Increase garlic
supplementation and add *Standardized Grapefruit Extract* (I
recommend Nutri-Biotic's *Citracidal*), *Astragalus*, *Echinacea*,
and/or *Golden Seal Root*. These are all excellent, safe, and
very effective natural antibiotics, which will work on the
source of the infection and stimulate the immune system.

A homeopathic remedy that promotes drainage or a
combination of remedies for infections can also be supportive in stimulating the body's defenses against the infection.
Remedies that work well include *Antimonium Crudum* for
skin infections with oozing and thick, yellow crusts, *Kal.
Mur.* and *Kal. Phos.* (two types of tissue cell salts that aid in
infections) or *Bioplasma* (the combination of all twelve tissue
cell salts) and *Arsenicum*.

Loss of appetite. First determine if there is any fever present. If there is, see recommendations under *Fever*. Feed up
to 100 mg. of *B-Complex vitamins* per day for cats or dogs.
Many multiple vitamin/mineral products already include B
vitamins, so check to see what you are already giving the
animal first. Try a few doses of homeopathic *Arsenicum* (in
general), *Nux Vomica* (if accompanied by one or more symptoms including nausea, vomiting, stool problems, flatulence) or *Belladonna* (if accompanied by nausea, empty
retching and vomiting, as well as an aversion to drinking). A
dose or two daily of any of the above remedies, especially
fifteen minutes prior to feeding, can also help stimulate
appetite. Several flower essences, especially a combination
formulation for minimizing stress, can often settle an animal

enough so that it begins to regain some appetite. Always address emotional stress when appetite loss is evident, as it can often be a contributing factor.

Skin eruptions are the most common of detoxification symptoms. *Horsetail* and *Milk Thistle* are excellent herbs to use at this time, but homeopathic remedies such as *Apis* or *Sepia* (dry, rashly skin), *Rhus Tox.* (for clusters of tiny pimples that are extremely itchy), or *Graphites* (for scabby, oozy eruptions) work quickly to relieve irritation and discomfort. When in doubt try a dose of *Arsenicum* or *Sulphur*, both general skin remedies. *Antimonium Crudum* is best when staphylococcal or streptococcal infections are also present in the skin. Follow the above recommendations for infections as well.

Vomiting can also lead to dehydration and is often strictly symptomatic of detoxification rather than being an attempt to rid the stomach of an irritant. Therefore, since persistent vomiting will quickly exhaust your pet, it is appropriate to suppress this symptom quickly. Homeopathy works well, and is easier to administer, because it won't cause vomiting as an herb would. For vomiting after eating, a combination of *Arsenicum* and *Nux Vomica* is effective. When vomiting occurs after drinking, use *Phosphorus* (with or without *Arsenicum*). Give one dose of each, every fifteen minutes for the first hour, then one dose every hour, until there has been no more vomiting for one hour. (See "Symptoms A to Z.")

PROPER NUTRITION

The primary line of defense to prevent or treat any degenerative disorder is a sound nutritional program. After detoxification is a perfect time to introduce a healthier diet.

Your pet's natural diet should consist of fresh, high-quality, easy to digest and assimilate ingredients. Since home cooking is optimal, but not very practical for many people, you should seek a quality commercial product. Become an educated label reader, look beyond catchy terms such as "senior diet," "low protein," "organic," "natural," and "human-grade quality," and ask the manufacturer directly to prove the quality of their products and guarantee their formula.

Seek only Grade A or B meats (human grade) and avoid the four-D meats—dead, dying, diseased, or disabled animals not fit for human consumption. Four-D meats are those most commonly used in pet foods.

Grain by-products are prevalent, problematic ingredients in commercial pet products. These include wheat millings, brewer's rice (waste from brewing), and flours. These inexpensive fillers are not only devoid of nutritional value, but can also severely compromise your pet's health. Manufacturers often include rancid and moldy grains in their products because they are cheaper. These poor-quality grain by-products increase the possibility of a toxic reaction. Only Grade 1 or 2 grains (human grades) should be used, preferably whole ground, to ensure that their nutritional goodness remains intact.

People are often concerned that changing their pet's diet will result in digestive upsets. This is true only if you are changing from a poor-quality or chemical-based diet to another one of the same quality. When you switch to a healthier, more natural diet, there should be no irritating ingredients to upset the balance. The only problems your pet might have are soft stool and gas. This may happen because you may be overfeeding your pet with the new diet.

One cup of a grocery-store food is almost fifty percent filler! A better brand of grocery-type foods, even pet shop pet food, or prescription diets can be just as bad. These may have less filler, but they will probably contain other types of by-products, which may alter the volume of nutrients available in one cup. When switching to a higher-quality food, there generally is less filler, and therefore, feeding the same quantities (cup for cup) would result in overfeeding of the better brand. Carefully read and follow the manufacturer's recommendations for the food, and watch your pet carefully for the first few weeks to see how they react.

Overfeeding can often occur when people begin to cook for their pets. It is difficult to recommend one recipe that will suit everybody's needs, so I suggest that you seek out a well-researched book on natural pet care that includes recipes.

Beware of feeding your pet raw meats, which can upset, rather than support your pet's condition. I believe this is because animals adapt to fit their environment. Our pets have been domesticated for so long that they have been altered to become processed food eaters and have lost the wild animal's ability to digest raw meat tissue, bone, hide, feathers, etc., on a regular basis. Even if you give your pet a digestive enzyme, your pet will probably have to struggle to digest raw animal tissue.

If you prefer home-cooked foods to commercially processed pet foods, and you will lightly cook the food so that all the enzymes and nutrients are not destroyed, cooking will break down the meat sufficiently, making it easier for your pet's digestive tract to handle.

Even with the best-quality and balanced diet (commercial or home-cooked), nutritional supplementation is necessary to provide many nutrients now missing from our food chain. For instance, research indicates that fifty years ago spinach had up to eighty percent more nutritional value than today. This is true in varying degrees for other vegetables, grains, and fruits, as well as meats from animals fed "off the land." Our earth has been stripped of many of the naturally occurring micronutrients found in soil, which are then assimilated by plants. Years of overfarming, using toxic chemicals or fertilizers, and environmental pollution (such as acid rain) have taken its toll.

Even organic farming methods cannot guarantee that the produce is more nutritious, as it will take approximately seventy-five years of organic farming before these nutrients are returned to the soil. Therefore, it is important that we supplement our animals' diets to ensure that they receive the fundamental nutrients required. Even pet foods which are "nutritionally complete" according to AAFCO (American Association of Feed Control Officers) still may not provide all that is needed for basic good health. For instance, the AAFCO standards require a certain amount of protein per cup of food, but that protein does not have to be digestible. So what good is it? This is also true for certain sources of Vitamin A or calcium, among other nutrients.

Proper nutrition not only includes quality, easy to digest foods, but also appropriate supplementation to support health. Such a regime will stimulate your pet's curative potential, and also increase the ability to reverse any adverse symptom.

KEY INGREDIENTS FOR A HEALTHY DIET

- Fresh ingredients that do not have an unpleasant odor due to rancidity
- Whole foods such as whole ground grains, not "flours," "mill runs," or "by-products"

- Concentrated protein sources known as "meal" (as in "lamb meal" or "beef meal") are preferred over whole meats (listed only as "lamb"). This is not to be confused with "by-product meal."

"Meal" refers to the process of removing up to eighty percent, but no less than forty-five percent, of the ingredient's water content. There is more meat protein for your money, since water only adds to the weight of the ingredients. Weight is listed on the product label by the heaviest to lightest ingredient. It is deceiving to find chicken (or turkey, rabbit, fish, and other animal sources) listed first, when the majority of protein is coming from grains, not animal protein. The cost of the product is considerably less when a protein other than an animal protein is used. One pound of meal is equivalent to approximately three pounds of whole meat, and since there is an additional charge to dehydrate the meat, many companies use the meat to draw you to the label, but use a cheaper ingredient for the actual protein—a protein source that could trigger arthritic symptoms.

Look for identifiable and digestible animal protein or fat sources such as beef, beef meal, lamb, lamb meal, lamb fat, chicken, chicken meal or chicken fats, turkey, ostrich, etc., not vague terms like "meats," "poultry by-product meal," or "animal fats."

Look for *USDA Grade A or B animal protein sources*, preferably raised without growth hormones or recently given antibiotics (possible with some free-range raised lamb, cattle, or chicken).

Look for *USDA Grade 1 or 2 whole grains*, preferably free of chemical pesticides or herbicides. Organic grains are not cost-effective for use in commercial pet foods yet (if your pet's food claims "organic," demand written certification), but "pesticide-free" or "washed grains" are available. If you are cooking for your pet, buy the best you can afford!

Balanced, combined protein and grain sources suit most pets better than single source ingredients, contrary to popular belief. Vegetable and fruit fiber should be present, such as carrots and apples, for proper digestion, natural flavoring, and trace nutrients. Fiber is important to elimination, and is full of nutrients when additionally provided in whole grains. Quality sources of fat are necessary for energy and good coats. Vegetable or fish oils should be used, rather than animal fats. Because cats have a higher metabolism than dogs, they need the higher fat content, and high-quality animal fats are acceptable.

Price. Often, the cheaper foods are actually more expensive, meal to meal, because you have to feed so much more than a better-quality diet, with less filler.

Product should be fresh when purchased. Check the manufacture date, not the expiration date. Manufacturers will never admit the food won't really last a year. Never feed your pet food, especially naturally preserved food, that is older than six months, unless it has a completely sealed, airtight, barrier bag. Stale food not only doesn't taste good, it has lost most of its nutritional value through oxidation, and the ingredients are no longer as bio-available.

INGREDIENTS TO AVOID IN A HEALTHY DIET

Foul-smelling ingredients should be avoided at all cost. No matter what the date is on the bag, smell it when you open the bag and if it smells rancid, don't feed it to your pet.

Greasy food. If you see oil on the bag or on the cans of pet food, it is high in animal fats or tallow. These can include rendered carcasses and recycled cooking grease from restaurants. These fats are difficult to digest and often rancid prior to the manufacturing process.

Animal by-products such as "beef by-product," "lamb by-product," "chicken by-product" are a mixture of the whole carcass including feces, cancerous tumors, hide, hooves, beaks, feathers, and fur. "Meat" or "meat by-products" are a mixture of whatever mammals, including road kill, rats, and other dogs and cats ground together. "Poultry by-products" are a mixture of whatever feathered animals, including pigeons, ground together, and should definitely not be fed to your pet.

Grain by-products such as "mill runs," "flours," "middlings," "husks," and "parts" should be avoided at all costs. They have no nutritional value because all available nutrients have been removed in the manufacturing process. They may be harsh on an animal's digestive and eliminatory tracts, and irritate the body as it attempts to process them. These cheap fillers are used as additional protein sources to increase the finished product's weight and mass, although they are non-digestible and therefore cannot be assimilated.

Fillers such as powdered "cellulose" and "cellulose fiber" can include recycled newspaper, sawdust, and cardboard. "Plant cellulose" is usually ground peanut hulls—which are very damaging to sensitive colon tissues. Beet pulp or grain by-products have no significant nutritional value, but do add bulk and weight to the finished product.

Yeast is a cheap source of B vitamins, amino acids, and some nutrients. Touted for flea control and energy, yeast can contribute to allergies by burdening the liver and interfering in proper digestion.

Sugar is added to most commercial diets and treats. On pet food labels it can be called "sucrose," "beet pulp," "molasses," "cane syrup," "fruit solids," and of course, "sugar." It is a very cheap, heavy filler (cost effective for the manufacturer) and is also addictive (the pet will want more of the same). Additional sugar in the diet is the primary cause of weight problems and diabetic conditions, both of which make arthritic conditions worse.

Symptom Reversal

Once you have established a good foundation by detoxification and proper diet so that the body can draw strength to fuel its curative process, it is time to address the individual needs of your pet. Although the basic curative process is the same for all living beings, each one of us has our own unique journey toward symptom reversal.

All of our symptoms have a history, unique to our own experiences. A youthful body can cope with a multitude of stresses and maintain some balance, but as the body grows older and becomes more burdened as its biological processes naturally begin to slow down, it can become overwhelmed by its lifestyle.

The history of disease and the curative process is determined by the age of the pet, how genetically compromised they are, the quality of their lifestyle, and the severity and duration of the symptoms. I have never seen an animal that was too old, too weak, too young, too sick, or too hopeless to respond to holistic animal care. Is every case a complete success? That depends on your definition of success. Every animal's symptoms, when addressed holistically, experience some positive change.

Seventy-five percent of pets respond immediately to detoxification and nutritional support, and a high number experience long-term symptom reversal. Fifteen percent need additional naturopathic (including acupuncture or acupressure, chiropractic, and massage), plus homeopathic and/or herbal support, to complete the curative process and effectively reverse their structural disease.

Eight percent of pets might need some medical or chemical support: short-term symptom suppression through pain medication (when arthritis is severely damaging the pet's overall health) and steroids (when lack of mobility is life-threatening). Many of these animals can benefit from short-term support until the natural support they are receiving takes over. Unfortunately, probably half of these animals were given chemicals because the body's attempts to rebalance were misunderstood. Classic symptoms of detoxification were visible, but the owner or veterinarian arrested the process with medical treatment. Some of these owners later returned to detoxification successfully, but others remained in the cycle of symptom suppression for years before they allowed the detoxification process to be completed. Others simply gave up.

Two percent of suffering pets will always have arthritis regardless of what is done. Symptoms can be suppressed holistically and/or chemically for short-term relief, but as soon as treatment is stopped, the cycle begins anew. These pets are either too genetically compromised or too overwhelmed by their condition to ever successfully reverse their disease on their own. Remember that the more holistic the lifestyle, the easier it will be to keep the pet's resistance to toxins high and their biological functions processing to their fullest potential—even if you choose to use medication as well. Each year your pet lives a holistic lifestyle, its body will continue to strengthen, and many symptoms will become easier to handle, or even eventually reverse themselves. Detoxification also protects the liver, kidneys, and other vital organs from toxic drug side effects. At the very least, holistic animal care can slow the degenerative process.

Zaezar, my fourteen-year-old female Rottweiler, has a genetic predisposition to hip dysplasia. Because she was raised on natural diets and looked so healthy, I had become lax in her supplement regime. She developed symptoms around five years ago, and her mobility was so compromised at times that we were forced to limit her daily activity. We addressed her structural weaknesses holistically, and this year she needed fewer doses of her herbal anti-inflammatory because she is so much stronger! Once again, she enjoys wandering the property. She is a prime example of the fact that even in older, genetically compromised pets, through adhering to a holistic lifestyle and supporting symptoms—even if temporary suppression is needed—positive change can occur.

Common sense is the most valuable tool you possess for reversing arthritic symptoms. Ask yourself if what you are doing is getting you the results you want. If not, re-evaluate, but do continue addressing the problem. Not doing something is *not* an option. *Nothing comes from nothing.* On countless occasions, people exclaim, "I thought I'd just wait and see if it got any better on its own." They are shocked that the condition gets worse! By the time they get around to doing something, it may be too late, the body too weakened, or the dis-ease too deep, and it is so much harder to regain balance!

The only time that it is appropriate to do nothing is during detoxification or a curative response, where the health of the animal may temporarily become worse as the body attempts to rebalance itself. To do something (to suppress) during this time only stops the process, and drives the imbalance deeper into the body.

It is appropriate to address symptoms through holistic animal care when:

- Any non-life-threatening symptom has been present for four to eight hours.
- There are acute (sudden) symptoms from over-exertion or toxins: stiffness, digestive upset, discharges, irritations, pustules,

irritability or emotional stress, including withdrawal (often the results of exhaustion due to pain).

- There are acute flare-ups of chronic (ongoing) symptoms, especially during detoxification.
- Known triggers are present, such as during high-exertion days. Many of my arthritic symptom reversal suggestions can also be applied as a preventative.
- A curative response has been ongoing for more than forty-eight hours.

It is appropriate to address symptoms through allopathic, veterinary care when:

- There is any life-threatening acute symptom, especially paralysis, respiratory difficulties resulting in hyper-panting, an excessive heart rate present for two to four hours, loss of consciousness, excessive dehydration, or uncontrollable shaking.
- High fever is present for more than twenty-four hours.
- Chronic symptom aggravation for more than twenty-four hours results in loss of mobility, uncontrollable digestive upsets, urinary dysfunction, or other severe symptoms.
- Unmanageable infectious states, even if mild, have lasted for four to six weeks.

When in doubt, seek out a trusted professional to support your pet's process.

HELPFUL HINTS

Feed a high-quality diet and supplement at least twice per day— more often if needed to help stabilize blood sugar, support the immune system, and reduce the arthritic reaction.

Supplement with the proper nutrients, including glandular products and herbs, for a strong foundation from which to stimulate the body's curative response.

Remember, it can take three to six weeks for detoxification and increased assimilation of nutrients to begin establishing the necessary foundation for a successful curative process. During this time old cells are being replaced with the newer, healthier cells, which will bring change to the overall condition. Therefore, it is best to allow the body some time to respond on its own before adding too many other ingredients to the mix. Provide a high-quality multiple vitamin and mineral supplement with basic herbal or homeopathic support for the first month or two, until you better understand the specific underlying imbalance. Remember that approximately eight out of ten pets successfully reverse their arthritis with this alone. Additional supplements or medications may overwhelm the body with ingredients it doesn't need and interfere with the body's natural curative process. Explore each product available to see what is specifically recommended in your situation. Be sure to read ingredient labels carefully, and follow all instructions listed on any products you choose to use on your animals.

Utilize homeopathy to help maximize the body's curative potential, especially the processes of detoxification and symptom reversal.

Homeopathy is safe to use in addition to herbs or medications, although drugs may interfere with a remedy's healing potential. To utilize homeopathic remedies to their fullest potential, follow a few simple suggestions. Homeopathy is very helpful in reducing acute flare-ups and supports symptom reversal on a deeper level than herbs or supplements alone. Homeopathy can often be the key to reversing a deeper acute or chronic weakness. Although a lot of emphasis is placed on potencies, I have found many to be successful in a wide range of potencies, so I am more inclined to support getting what is available to you, whether it is a 6X and not a 3C. For the majority of acute reactions, even if due to chronic conditions, utilizing the lower potencies will effect change. These potencies range anywhere from 3X to

30C. For long-term reversal of a specific disorder, utilizing the higher 200C potency will be effective, after lower potencies have brought the acute reaction under control. High potencies, such as Ms, should be used with professional guidance. By giving the body a boost with homeopathic remedies, other supplements will act more quickly and effectively.

When beginning a homeopathic remedy, I recommend building up its action in the body through frequent dosing. You can not overdose your pet. Give one dose orally, according to the manufacturer's recommendations, every fifteen minutes for the first hour, then every hour until there is relief. To maintain relief, dose a minimum of twice daily for an additional one to two weeks. More frequent dosing may be administered as needed. Resume homeopathic treatment or any another appropriate remedy whenever the symptom presents itself, and follow this schedule until there is complete reversal. Long-term maintenance is also possible through a weekly dose of the most beneficial remedy.

I prefer liquid remedies because they are easier to give. If the dropper touches your hands or your pet, rinse it off before returning to the bottle. Most remedies come in sugar pellets (use as is) or tablets (crush inside a piece of paper first for best application). To avoid contamination and a reduction in efficacy, do not handle these remedies with your bare hands. Rather, use the cap or a clean piece of paper to administer the dose. Always allow at least fifteen minutes between food or strong extracts when giving homeopathic remedies.

Use synergistic modalities such as chiropractic care, massage, touch, and energy therapies, including giving acupressure therapy at home in-between veterinary acupuncture sessions. Home therapy will prolong the benefits received in a clinical visit.

Maintain a Holistic Animal Care lifestyle, even in-between reactions, to help enhance the body's defenses and further balance the body's weaknesses. With each month the body will continue to gain balance and strength, including joint support and resistance to general sensitivities known to trigger inflammation. Remember, symptom suppression—even holistically but without constitutional support—only leads to a reoccurrence of symptoms, not a long-term reversal of dis-ease.

Injury-proof your home by removing obstacles to free mobility for older or arthritis-prone pets. Arthritic reactions are often caused by a physical stress on the weakened joints. This is common to pets who struggle up and down furniture, stairs, and uneven terrain. If the floor is too slippery, causing your pet fall and twist its legs, use some throw rugs with a rubber backing for better footing. If the bed or couch is too high, try a stool or carpet-covered box next to it for your pet to get on first. Don't take your pet on difficult hikes, allow them to ride in the back of a pickup truck or anywhere their footing is unstable. Avoid forcing your pet to struggle; this will relieve much of their discomfort and avoid chronic damage to the joints and ligaments.

Provide support for weakened joints to relieve pain and slow the degenerative process. Feed and water your pet off the floor at shoulder height to minimize stress on the neck and back. Provide a firm, foam pad rather than a fluffy bed that may be harder to get out of. A pillow or folded up towel under the head can provide relief by supporting the neck in the proper position when your pet is sleeping.

Another thing to consider is helping the partially paralyzed or immobile pet to get around. Maintaining some type of mobility is vital to supporting a curative response. Cats and smaller dogs can be carried and helped by hand.

This can be very difficult for some owners when the dog is large or the owner is limited in his or her abilities. The use of a sling can give the pet a sense of security and help the owner handle the load. A sling can be purchased, or made by wrapping a towel around the midsection and grasping the top as a handle. For extremely large dogs you can use two people with two towels. Always be careful not to interfere with the movement of the legs or the ability to breathe. This technique relieves some of the weight on the joints and stabilizes the pet on its feet so that it can walk. For the paralyzed pet, wheelchair-designed braces are available.

Exercise can help or damage the pet further depending on how far you stress the joint. Swimming is the best form of strengthening and increasing the range of motion in arthritic joints. If walking is the only option, limit exercise to several smaller walks rather than one or two longer ones. Massage your pet and help them stretch for a few minutes before and after exercise. Never force your pet to go farther than they are telling you they can. Animals simply do not fake pain.

Animals can injure themselves because they are compelled to keep up with their pack leader. They become excited at the prospect of going for a walk or a car ride and their enthusiasm can make them push themselves beyond the point of damage. You must carefully monitor your pet's activity and slow them down when needed to prevent aggravating their condition.

Do not underestimate the power of nature; recognize that nature can take longer to suppress a symptom than a drug, but often will do the job more completely.

Support the curative power of nature and avoid interfering with it. Use chemicals and medications carefully. Avoid vaccinations whenever possible.

Use common sense. Address changes in your animal's health or behavior as soon as possible, and pay attention to what your pet's symptoms are telling you. For example, if your dog's stiffness increases the day after you play with him, don't encourage his tugging on a toy for so long or continue using the same Frisbee routine. Identify actions that cause discomfort and adjust your pet's lifestyle accordingly. Something as simple as keeping nails trimmed to relieve pressure on arthritic toes can increase your pet's chances of recovery. Don't be frightened to try something, you can always go back to the old way.

Don't sabotage the healing process by incorrectly utilizing diets, veterinarian-prescribed medications, or natural supplement products. Read the directions. Ask questions! The more you know and understand, the more successful you will be.

Symptoms A to Z

This chapter lists the most common symptoms associated with arthritis, as well as some that are not commonly associated with structural imbalance, but which I suspect are related. Your pet may be experiencing a slightly different symptom than what I describe. Please try to match your particular needs as closely as possible to one of the symptoms listed. Be sure to have specific diagnoses and treatments confirmed by your veterinarian.

Adrenal Malfunction is common in animals who are also exhibiting arthritic reactions, especially in conjunction with chronic skin conditions. Often, it can actually be caused by previous cycles of steroid treatments, which are commonly used to suppress inflammatory symptoms. You may want to ask your veterinarian to consider testing for hormonal or cortisol levels. This will benefit you, no matter what you decide to do. If nothing has seemed to work, utilize any medication that is appropriate for you and your animal. Pets who have not responded well to natural modalities are often diagnosed with deeper glandular malfunctions, which, when addressed naturally, help stimulate the curative process.

There are many wonderful, natural glandular products available. I prefer *glandulars in powder or tablet form* to homeopathic ones, but do not disregard a homeopathic remedy combined with a potentized glandular *in addition* to a tableted form. Homeopathic glandulars work on a deeper level and are beneficial to overall support, whereas tableted glandulars actually feed the gland directly, providing more substantial support in reversing glandular weakness. *Multi-glandulars*, a combination of several glands, are beneficial in supporting the weaker gland, but make sure the combination contains sufficient amounts of the particular gland you need to stimulate and support. Add another single glandular product to the multiple, if needed. (See Cushing's Disease.)

Aggression can be a problem in pets suffering from arthritis. More commonly dietary ingredients themselves, especially sugars and chemical preservatives, contribute to the sensitivities and arthritic reaction, as well as trigger the aggression. In addition, some animals cannot tolerate the constant irritation caused by arthritis—exhausted from discomfort, they lash out when approached.

Also avoid stress, sudden movements, and abrupt awakening of the pet. These tend to trigger an outburst. Be sure that you are using *higher potencies of Vitamin B1, B2, and B6*: 50 mg. to 100 mg. for cats and dogs regardless of size, and B12: 50 mcg. to 125 mcg. for cats and dogs. Also use the homeopathic remedy *Aconite* for sudden or intense fear or *Ignatia* for grief and anger. Several flower essences such as *Chicory, Holly, Impatiens, Rock Rose*, and *Vine*, can also be helpful, as well as additional exercise. *Bryonia* is helpful when the slightest movement seems painful to your pet, and the aggression may be based in part to a pain response. Many aggressive pets have noticeable improvements in their dispositions shortly after the detoxification process.

Allergic Reactions are common in pets who also suffer from arthritis. Arthritis may be the symptom of an allergy. In general, allergies can be successfully suppressed with a few doses of homeopathy in lower potencies (3X to 30C).

Homeopathic Remedies for Allergic Reactions

- *Arsenicum* is an excellent remedy for arthritis and is also used for general irritations, hot spots, digestive imbalances, or toxicity.

- *Sulphur* is used for a wide variety of skin conditions, associated with intense itching, which become worse at night in warm surroundings. Scratching may seem to satisfy the pet temporarily, but often will result in increased itching and burning. *Sulphur* is also good for greasy skin. This remedy is well suited to pets with autoimmune disorders.

- *Apis* is good for intensely itchy skin that is aggravated by warmth, including the warmth the body may give off when covered in rashes. Joints are swollen and hot.

- *Rhus Tox* is helpful when the animal is rubbing or scratching its skin, when the animal gets wet, or cold weather seems to aggravate itchy skin. It is especially good for irritations around the head. Often this pet will have ligament problems.

- *Urtica Urens* addresses extensive eruptions, hives, or welts that are very itchy. Usually the skin is dry and aggravated by warmth or bathing. (These conditions are non-responsive to *Apis* or *Sulphur*.) It is also good for profuse discharges from mucous membranes. Symptoms may be localized to the right side of the body.

- *Sabadilla* is a popular hay-fever remedy, addressing common upper-respiratory symptoms such as asthma, spasmodic sneezing, watery nasal discharge, facial itching, irritated ears and red, and runny eyes.

- *Euphrasia* is another excellent remedy for allergy-related eye and tear duct irritations.

- *Nux Vomica* addresses the majority of digestive imbalances, including gas, vomiting, diarrhea, or lack of appetite, especially when dosed with *Arsenicum*.

Herbal antihistamines and anti-inflammatory products are very effective and a good alternative to over-the-counter drugs, such as *Benadryl*® "or veterinary prescriptions, such as *Prednisone*. I recommend that you use a combination of homeopathy for acute reaction and herbs to lessen sensitivity, which may reduce a more severe reaction.

Herbs for Allergic Reactions

- *Yucca Root* has been used for centuries by indigenous cultures to reduce general inflammation. Current studies have confirmed that bio-available steroidal saponins (found mostly in pure extract form, rather than the fibrous powder that is a waste product of extraction) perform as effectively as their chemical counterparts (steroids such as *Prednisone*) without the serious drug side effects. *Yucca* enhances the action of other, more specific-use herbs, in working more effectively by supporting organ function and detoxification.

- *Chinese Ephedra* is a powerful antihistamine, which quickly reduces inflammation. This herb has been abused as a stimulant, but it is very safe when used as directed. *Ephedra* reduces the itching of a histamine response and can be used for both topical (eyes, ears, skin) and internal (irritable bowels, inflamed respiratory passages) symptoms.

- *Marshmallow* and/or *Bayberry Root* reduces inflammation in general, and is helpful with detoxification of histamine and in reducing respiratory stress.

- *Eyebright Herb* helps address general allergy symptoms affecting the eyes.

- *Stinging Nettle Leaf* reduces general redness and irritation of the skin, eyes, and ears. It can also help reduce irritation of the anal glands and is good for swollen joints.

- *Red Clover Blossoms* are useful in reversing skin eruptions, as well as reducing coughs and bronchitis. It eliminates free radicals that inflame joints and is an immune stimulant.

- *Eyebright, Bayberry Root Bark, Golden Seal Root, Calamus*, and *Stinging Nettle Leaf* function together to contract swollen mucous membranes associated with hay fever and allergies. Their anti-bacterial properties help keep infections of the eyes and ears in check. Several of these herbs help reverse joint inflammation as well.

- *Turmeric Root, Black Catechu, Grindelia Floral Buds*, and *Lobelia*, combined, protect the liver from circulating antigens and allergens, thereby reducing infections and skin or intestinal irritations associated with airborne and food-related allergies. This combination supports the adrenal glands when epinephrine is needed by the body during inflammatory responses generated by allergens. It also is indicated for all disorders of hypersensitivity, including allergies, asthma, dermatitis, irritable bowel syndrome, and food-related digestive disorders. Reduces sciatic or joint edema and toxemia. Helps eliminate free radicals responsible for joint deterioration.

Appetite Problems, especially loss of appetite, can occur during curative responses, particularly when your animal is in pain. First, be sure there is no fever present, and that your pet is not dehydrated, which is a more serious problem. (See Fever and Infection.) Also determine the level of stress your pet may be experiencing and address that, as stress can also interfere with appetite. (See Behavioral Problems.)

For nutritional support, feed up to 100 mg. of B-Complex vitamins per day. This, in addition to a short fast, can quickly stimulate the appetite. Often, a lack of appetite is the result of a toxic overload. Be sure to question any medications your pet is taking.

Try a few doses of homepathic *Arsenicum* for general appetite loss; *Nux Vomica* when appetite loss is accompanied by one or more symptoms including nausea, vomiting, stool problems, flatulence; or *Belladonna* with mostly nausea, empty retching and vomiting as well as an aversion to drinking. A dose or two daily, *especially fifteen minutes prior to feeding*, can also help stimulate appetite. Several flower essences, especially *Mimulus, Star of Bethlehem*, and *Rock Rose*, or a combination, can often settle an animal enough so that it begins to regain an appetite.

Arthritis is an inflammatory reaction in the joints or spine and is often used as a catch-all phrase to identify a wide variety of symptoms associated with muscle, bone, and joint disorders. These symptoms are generally a flare-up in conjunction with, or as a direct reaction to, certain physical conditions, especially involving congested or malfunctioning livers, kidneys, pancreases, adrenal, and thyroid glands.

Symptoms can best be prevented or suppressed and possibly eventually reversed homeopathically and/or herbally while the structure (joints, ligaments, muscles, and tendons) is strengthened through nutritional supplementation.

Homeopathic Remedies for Arthritis

- *Arsenicum* is an excellent general homeopathic arthritic remedy, especially for reactive or infectious arthritis.
- *Arnica* reduces swelling, general muscular pain, and discomfort. *Arnica* is an excellent preventative remedy when used prior to, and during, exertion.
- *Bryonia* helps when the pet is stiff upon standing and *cannot* walk out of it.
- *Rhus Tox* is for the pet that is stiff upon standing but *can* walk out of it.
- *Hypericum* reduces nerve irritation and pain in animals who are constantly licking their legs and feet, and even their backs. Use with *Ruta* for intervertebral disc disorders. *Hypericum* helps address paralysis; slows paralytic deterioration.
- *Ruta* is best for severe tendon or ligament strains, common in nutritionally depleted pets. It helps repair Cruciate (knee), hip, shoulder, and intervertebral ligaments, often eliminating the need for surgery, and stabilizes degenerative disorders like Wobbler's.
- *Apis* helps when joints are visibly swollen, tender to the touch, and hot. This pet prefers to stay cool.
- *Causticum* is indicated for painful chronic arthritic or paralytic afflictions including joint deformities with progressive loss of muscular strength and coordination.

- *Carbo Veg.* is used for the older pet that may be overweight and who displays a lack of circulation indicated by cold extremities or mouth. This pet moves slowly with heavy feet that seem paralyzed. The joints are very weak, and this pet feels worse at night when the air is damp.
- *Gelsemium* helps hip dysplasia; when pain is localized to the lumbar and sacral region including the lower extremities and the back muscles are very tight.
- *Colchicum* addresses symptoms due to a lack of synovial fluid and marked muscular tension, especially when body is humped in pain. It is best for shifting pains.
- *Dulcamara* is beneficial for cold, damp weather-reactive arthritis, not responsive to *Bryonia* or *Rhus*. It is also indicated for acute flare-ups that border on paralysis.
- *Strychninum* is indicated for rheumatic pain from stiff limbs and joints. Limbs may twitch or shake and muscular spasms occur suddenly. Panting from pain is common.
- *Symphytum* addresses injuries to the tendons and periosteum, and neuralgia of knees. It is an excellent remedy for chronic Cruciate damage resulting in arthritis.
- *Gaultheria* is best for generalized rheumatism and neuralgia.
- *Calcarea Phos.* is a tissue cell salt that lessens the tendency towards over-calcification. It is beneficial for the arthritic pet that hesitates going up steps or steps gingerly.
- *Bioplasma Tissue Cell Salts* are a combination of all twelve tissue-repairing cell salts. These help promote the assimilation of nutrients necessary for strengthening bone, tendon, muscles, or ligament tissues. It is especially beneficial for pets with structural disorders or "old age."

Herbal Supplements for Arthritis

- *Yucca* is a very effective anti-inflammatory. The stalk and roots contain steroidal saponins, which react in the body in a manner similar to chemical steroids without the side effects that chemical steroids produce. Saponins also reduce tissue inflammation and pain. Be sure to use a cold-pressed *Yucca* extract, rather than powder or tincture. The extract contains up to eighty-five percent more bio-available saponins and is easier on the digestive tract then other forms. It can be safely used with prescription steroids or painkillers.

- *Garlic*, naturally high in tissue-repairing properties, is a wonderful supplement for joints affected by toxic reactions, particularly infectious arthritis. Use highest allicin content possible and give 500 mg. to 1000 mg. per day for small dogs and cats, up to 2000 mg. for medium to large-sized dogs.
- *Milk Thistle, Siberian Ginseng, Licorice, Alfalfa*, and *Dandelion* are all excellent herbs for liver and blood detoxification, reducing free radicals that can irritate joints.
- *Hawthorn Berry* leaves and flowers contain bio-active flavonoids that stimulate connective tissue repair and strengthening. It enhances the body's use of Vitamin C.
- *Licorice Root* and *White Willow Bark* are commonly used anti-inflammatories. Do not use *White Willow Bark* (aspirin) on cats, who can have a deadly reaction.

Nutritional Supplements for Arthritis

- *Vitamin C* helps reduce inflammation, strengthen ligaments and tendons to help stabilize joints, and reduces sensitivities to free radicals. Dose to bowel tolerance or at least 1000 mg. for cats and small dogs—up to 4000 mg. for larger dogs given in two daily doses.
- *MSM* is a sulfur-based product, which not only helps reduce inflammation and strengthen ligaments, but is also wonderful for poor skin and coat conditions.
- *Anti-oxidants*, such as *Grape Seed Extract* (50 mg. to 100 mg.) which is stronger than *Pycnogenol's Pine Bark*™, *Selenium* (15 mcg. to 50 mcg. per day), SOD (500 mg. to 1500 mg. per day), and Vitamin E (75 IU to 150 IU per day), reverse inflammation by reducing free radicals that can gather in and around joints triggering the inflammatory reaction. These also stimulate the immune system.
- *Shark Cartilage* and *Chondroitin Sulfates* provide mucopolysaccharides that benefit stiff joints by promoting synovial fluid lubrication. They also strengthen ligaments.

- *Glucosamines* help replenish synovial fluid, a shortage of which can create the rubbing of bone upon bone, resulting in pain and encouraging calcium build-up, which can result in more severe arthritis. Use at least 500 mg. to 1500 mg. per day, regardless of size. Each pet will have varying tolerances to this supplement, depending on the type of Glucosamines used. Glucosamine sulfate is a better choice than Glucosamine hydrochloride.
- One mg. to three mg. per day of *Boron* aids proper calcium absorption and strengthens bone density that is affected by metabolic bone disease or cancer. *Boron* helps the body avoid calcium build-up or over-calcification, common in arthritic conditions. (See Structural Disorders.)

Autoimmune Disease (See Immune System Dysfunction, Structural Disorders.)

Behavioral Problems are often associated with arthritic symptoms. Discomfort can trigger aggression, though some animals respond with nervousness, shyness, or complete withdrawal. Flower essences and homeopathic remedies work to address the underlying emotional aspect of most behavioral problems.

Flower Essences and Homeopathic Remedies for Behavioral Problems

- *Star of Bethlehem* is good for learned stresses. For example, if you overexerted your cat and your cat experienced pain after exertion, she may not trust you to be near her now.
- *Mimulus* is the remedy for minimizing fears of all types: fear of being massaged, fear of having ears or eyes cleaned, fear of wind and thunder, etc.
- *Rock Rose* is used for present terror. The body or muscles seem frozen.
- *Vine* is for the overbearing pet that demands attention.

- *Impatiens* quiets the pet that is always impatient and a little nervous, regardless of your reassurance.
- *Aconite* addresses behavior that is the result of situations that produced sudden shock or fear. It also addresses stiffness that becomes worse with emotional stress.
- *Pulsatilla* quiets the pet who wants to be held when in pain.
- *Ignatia* helps reduce symptoms related to grief or loss.

Unfortunately, nervousness, fear, or any intense emotion can reduce immune function and leave a pet very susceptible to reactive arthritis. Herbs such as *Valerian Root, Hops Flowers, Skullcap, Chamomile, St. John's Wort* (which also helps balance hormones) help to relax the pet, allowing them to rest more comfortably and sleep more deeply—all necessary for supporting the curative process. These herbs can also improve pain management and relax muscular tension. (See Aggression.)

Calcification of the bone tissue can occur due to injury (bone on bone) or abnormal calcium absorption. The body produces and localizes calcium to knit the weakness or damage to the bone. This can lead to over-calcification and arthritis. The spine can become fused, the back stiff, and the neck unable to bend correctly. Common to structural disorders, chronic calcification leads to immobilization of the joint. It is vital that you utilize a daily calcium, magnesium, and boron supplement to stimulate proper calcium utilization rather than calcification build-up. (See Structural Disorders: Metabolic Bone Disease.)

Cancer can often be the end result of a long-term bout with structural disorders, as an "arthritic" condition will often accompany the other distressing symptoms of cancer. Cancerous cells can easily infect bone and demand so much energy from the body that it will become very susceptible to toxins. Unfortunately, I have seen many immune system problems, including Feline Leukemia, Feline Infectious Peritonitis (FIP), Tick Fever, Valley Fever, and chronic anemia (a possible pre-cancerous state), in pets originally diagnosed and treated chemically for "arthritis." I believe that the constant stress of arthritic reactions on the body, as well as the chemicals and drugs used to treat them, weakens the animal's constitution and their curative potential, as well as encourages damaged cells to become cancerous.

Many of the arthritic relief recommendations in this book are applicable to the treatment of cancerous conditions. In both cases (arthritic conditions and cancer), the underlying imbalance is likely to be in the immune system, and arthritis or cancer is the symptom. (See Immune System Dysfunction.)

Colitis and Irritable Bowel Syndrome are common secondary symptoms associated with arthritic conditions, especially with digestive innervation. Also, the constant stress of other arthritic symptoms, including pain, can also result in diarrhea, constipation (or alternating between the two), mucous-covered stools, flatulence, and even slight blood in the stool. *Nux Vomica* and *Arsenicum* are a good homeopathic combination to use initially. Digestive enzymes can also be appropriate, but I recommend that you limit their use to a few weeks at a time. The overuse of enzymes can cause additional digestive imbalance. Calming herbs, especially *Wild Oats* and *St. John's Wort*, are also helpful. Fiber supplementation with whole grain, fruit, and vegetables can provide proper evacuation and bowel care. *Yucca* is a wonderfully soothing herb, as is *Aloe* and *Slippery Elm Bark*. (See Constipation and Diarrhea.)

Constipation is a common symptom in arthritic pets. Whereas diarrhea is often associated with toxicity, alternating constipation and diarrhea, or constipation alone, can also occur because of underlying structural disorder. Constipation can weaken the body further because the waste products have not been properly eliminated and toxins will be reabsorbed from the colon into the bloodstream. Several factors can contribute to constipation, including pain medications like *Rymadal* and *Prednisone* often used for arthritis.

First eliminate any possible culprits:

- hard to digest pet food ingredients, such as "plant cellulose," often soy castings, peanut shells, or husks of any kind that are used as filler/fiber in pet food
- lack of exercise, when an animal has been confined for six hours or more
- inadequate fluid intake
- excessive ingestion of fur or hair, due to licking and chewing
- ingestion of non-digestible objects such as rocks, rubber, bones, or feathers
- poor sources of dietary fiber

Psyllium seed or husks are commonly used to regulate bowel movement, but, when used alone, often can be too harsh on the digestive tract. Combine psyllium with other fruits and vegetables like *carrots, apple fiber and pectin, guar gum* (a misunderstood, but excellent, source of natural fiber that swells to retain water), and *bran. Chinese mushrooms,* such as *Shiitake* and *Reishi,* which are also high in fiber, can help to reverse chronic colon conditions, including pre-cancerous growths. Cooked *oatmeal,* added to meals or given alone with vegetable, fish, or meat broth, not only is high in fiber, but also has detoxifying properties to help eliminate old fecal material from the bowels. (See Digestive Disorders.)

Cruciate Ligament (See Structural Disorders.)

Cushing's Disease is a serious malfunction of the adrenal gland, requiring a veterinarian's help. Many veterinarians have reported that, when adrenal malfunction is addressed holistically, symptoms of Cushing's Disease have also improved.

Symptoms can include fatigue, slow tissue repair, hair color loss or poor coat growth, excessive shedding, weak joints, and a droopy belly. (See Adrenal Malfunction.)

Degenerative Joint Disease (See Structural Disorders.)

Dermatitis often manifests in pets suffering from reactive arthritis because of the correlation between toxicity, the liver, and various symptoms. When the skin becomes irritated, inflamed, and itchy, pets begin to scratch, rub, chew, and lick themselves, and the skin becomes so irritated and inflamed that other problems arise: hair loss, dandruff, greasy skin, pimples, and hot spots.

A *hot spot* is an irritated, open area of skin caused by scratching or biting, which can result in infection. Keep the area dry and clean. Clip away the hair around the hot spot to make it easier to clean and treat topically. If a pet has chronic dermatitis and has been exposed to many cycles of antibiotics, a staphylococcal infection may arise that is difficult to treat.

Avoid the use of coal tar-based or chemically medicated shampoos. Do not bathe too often; when the skin is severely irritated, bathe no more than every two to four weeks. Spot cleaning and disinfecting can be done whenever needed. Over-frequent whole body bathing can worsen the condition by drying out the skin, thereby encouraging greasy skin. (Body oils will try to replenish themselves quickly and heavily to counter such drying.) Spot clean and disinfect the skin whenever needed.

Feed potent doses of a high quality *garlic* supplement (500 mg. to 1000 mg. per day for small dogs and cats, up to 2000 mg. for medium to large-sized dogs). In addition, other nutritional support for allergies, such as *Vitamin C*, will do more to clear up hot spots permanently, then topical treatment alone. (See Infections, Skin and Coat Problems.)

Diarrhea is often associated with drug allergies, although I have seen it in pets suffering from other stresses, especially constant tension and pain—all that nervous energy just churns up the bowel. *Psyllium seed or husk* is the most commonly used fiber to help regulate bowel movement, but often it can be too harsh on the digestive tract when used alone. Combine psyllium with other fruit and vegetable fiber sources such as *carrots, apple fiber and pectin, guar gum* (a misunderstood, but excellent, source of natural fiber that swells to retain water), and bran.

Chinese mushrooms, such as *Shiitake* and *Reishi*, have long been noted for their fiber content as well as their ability to reverse chronic colon conditions, including pre-cancerous growths, which may be irritated and triggering the diarrhea.

Cooked *oatmeal*, added to meals or given alone with vegetable, fish, or meat broth, is not only an excellent source of fiber, but also has detoxifying properties and can help eliminate old fecal material from the bowels. Old fecal material can become toxic (especially with bacterial infection) and can trigger the body's attempt to eliminate the irritation, resulting in the diarrhea.

Add to the oatmeal a high-quality garlic supplement (500 mg. to 1000 mg. per day for small dogs and cats, and up to 2000 mg. for medium to large-sized dogs). This regimen will give your pet natural antibiotic support.

These homeopathic remedies are effective in relieving diarrhea and associated symptoms. Use *Arsenicum* for general symptoms, *China* for debilitating fluid loss, and *Nux Vomica* for vomiting and/or appetite loss.

Herbally, use *Yucca* and/or *Calendula Extract*, *Liquid Chlorophyll*, and *Slippery Elm Extract or Powder* to soothe irritated intestinal tissues. Be sure that fluid intake is maintained, as diarrhea can quickly dehydrate your pet. Add one-half teaspoon of *raw honey* per twenty pounds of body weight per day to fluids or herbal preparations. Honey is not only soothing to an irritated colon, it is antiseptic and provides energy for a weakened pet. (See Digestive Disorders.)

Digestive Disorders are very common during curative responses, and can be associated with drugs and other environmental stresses. Lack of appetite, vomiting, stool changes, or flatulence often can accompany an arthritic episode. The use of digestive enzymes can be beneficial in the short term, but you will have to address the actual imbalance for long-term symptom reversal.

Homeopathic Remedies for Digestive Disorders

- *Arsenicum* is used for general digestive imbalances or toxicity and will alleviate most digestive disorders, especially if there is liver or spleen involvement, or if the disorder has been triggered by pain or anti-inflammatory medication.
- *Nux Vomica* also addresses the majority of digestive imbalances, including gas, vomiting, lack of appetite, or stool

problems (especially alternating between constipation and diarrhea). It complements *Arsenicum*.

- *Carbo Veg* is helpful when the pet is overweight, has chronic stool problems, seems to have trouble digesting well, and burps soon after eating. Is extremely beneficial when used with Nux Vomica, especially with senior pets.
- *Belladonna* is for the sudden onset of gastrointestinal symptoms that follow an arthritic episode. After initial use, it should be tapered off slowly and then followed by a more specific remedy.
- *Urtica Urens* addresses a lack of appetite often accompanied by extensive itchy eruptions, in addition to arthritis. These afflictions, which are not responsive to *Apis* or *Sulphur*, often appear in conjunction with digestive or eliminatory problems, and stiffness aggravated by warmth or resting.
- *Phosphorus* is indicated if the digestive problems include great debilitation, fluid loss, or frequent vomiting or diarrhea soon after meals. *Phosphorus* quickly eliminates blood (from old fecal material, viral, or bacterial detoxification) or fatty mucus (from pancreatic imbalance) in the stool.
- *Podophyllum* can be used when profuse, offensive-smelling stools occur. Color may be yellowish or greenish, is often completely liquid, or begins formed and turns loose as the bowel movement progresses, and can also be accompanied by dry heaves or gagging.
- *Pulsatilla* aids diarrhea or mucous-covered stools, which are often greenish in color. This stool will frequently change in character or color, even during the bowel movement. Diarrhea is likely to be worse at night or aggravated by warmth. Symptoms, such as nausea, vomiting, or diarrhea, are not too severe. Food might be vomited up partially digested. Nervous cats with generalized arthritic symptoms are particularly prone to these symptoms.
- *Bryonia* addresses those pets who are also cramping or whose stomachs rumble, but they avoid hard surfaces or respond in pain when their stomachs are rubbed. They may also exhibit arthritic pains as a result of an allergic reaction.

Herbal remedies can support reversal of many digestive upsets associated with arthritic reactions and can stabilize appetite. Many pets cannot tolerate herbs on an empty stomach. In fact, the herbs may create some of the digestive stress. When pets have digestive upsets, it is best to give herbs with a little food, until they are better tolerated, or you might try to obtain better-quality herbs. Encapsulate liquid extracts if needed.

Herbal Remedies for Digestive Disorders

- *Yucca Extract* provides natural steroidal saponins, which effectively reduce inflammation within the digestive system, including the stomach and intestinal lining as well as the liver, gall bladder, spleen, and pancreas. A reduction in excessive peristalsis (a squeezing response of the intestines to process and move digested material toward the colon) can help relieve diarrhea due to pain and inflammatory responses.
- *Garlic* is excellent for digestive complaints. Not only is it antiseptic and a natural antibiotic, it effectively supports proper digestion and colon health through its anti-parasitic and anti-yeast properties. High allicin content garlic supplements are beneficial in reversing general diarrhea, flatulence, and fatty stool deposits.
- *Peppermint Leaf* or *Fenugreek Seed* helps reduce intestinal gas, cramping, and colic, prevents fatty deposits, repairs digestive tissue ulcerations, and fights infection.
- *Dandelion Leaf* is an excellent tonic for the liver and gall bladder.
- *Siberian Ginseng Root* stimulates resistance against toxins, especially urea.
- *Milk Thistle Seed* supports proper liver function and detoxification.
- *Aloe* or *Calendula Extract* contain therapeutic components that soothe sensitive and irritated digestive tissues, including the stomach and intestinal lining, as well as the liver, gall bladder, spleen, and pancreas.

- *Devil's Club Root Bark, Indian Jambul Seed, Dandelion Leaf and Root, Uva Ursi Leaf,* and *Turmeric Root* reduce the occurrence of soft, fatty, off-colored stools due to pancreatic or blood sugar imbalance. This compound also slows rheumatoid arthritis.

- *Cascara Sagrada Bark, Barberry Root, Senna Leaves, Rhubarb Root,* and *Cayenne* clean out the intestinal tract. A detoxified colon is fundamental to re-balancing the digestive system and increasing the assimilation of nutrients necessary for proper health. These herbs can also prevent or reverse parasitic infestation.

- *Fennel Seed, Ginger Root,* and *Anise Seed* relieve gas, cramping, and mucus while stimulating proper digestion and peristalsis.

- *Shiitake* and *Reishi Mushrooms* have been used by the Chinese for centuries to prevent and treat cancers associated with the digestive system. Colon cancer in particular responds well to their incredible healing properties. A dramatic reduction in food sensitivities is often the result of long-term supplementation. (See Appetite Problems, Constipation, Colitis, Diarrhea.)

Ear Problems commonly occur in pets who suffer from toxicity and can be secondary symptoms to arthritis. The liver, a primary organ often affected by toxins, has a relationship to the ears and eyes. As the liver becomes burdened, the ears begin to exhibit symptoms associated with toxicity problems, often becoming more prone to irritation from free radicals, as well as foods and chemicals, prior to or during an arthritic episode.

Ears can be effectively cleaned with a homemade solution of two ounces of distilled or purified water, one teaspoon *Witch Hazel*, one teaspoon white vinegar, and six drops of *Calendula Extract* (add an additional six drops of *Golden Seal Extract*—if infection is suspected). Use a cotton ball to squeeze a little of this solution into the ear. Rub the outer base of the ear to massage the solution into any debris that needs to be removed (you may hear a slight suction-like noise inside the ear). Allow your pet to shake out their ears, then wipe out the rest of debris and fluid with a soft tissue wrapped around your finger. To avoid damage, do not insert anything down into the inner ear, but rather let the tissue absorb any impurities. Follow cleaning with an application of *Calendula Extract*, *Aloe Gel* or *Vitamin E*. Use *Hypericum*, *Calendula*, or *Arnica Cream* around the flap and opening, if pain is present.

Be careful not to use heavy, oil-based ingredients or vegetable oils. Although such oils may seem to be conditioning the ear and reducing irritation, they may also be nurturing a bacterial or yeast infection, by providing a warm, moist, oxygen-less environment. For dogs with ear flaps in the down position, tie them up over the head with an elastic hair band to encourage air circulation. As little as one hour of air circulation per day can reduce bacterial or yeast growth, and encourage healing.

Grapefruit Extract ear drops can also be applied after cleaning the ear to fight bacterial and yeast infections. *Mullein* and *Garlic Oil* ear drops are also excellent for irritated and infected ears.

Avoid alcohol-based products, which can irritate the ears further—unless you suspect water is trapped in the ear channel, in which case a few drops of pure alcohol can dry up the fluid residue. Don't worry about the alcohol found in herbal extracts—very little alcohol remains by the final dilution.

Herbal Remedies for Ear Problems

- *Garlic* is vital to eliminating ear problems. Use a high-potency supplement for basic antibacterial support. Because it is high in natural sulfur, garlic helps heal damaged tissue.

- *Yucca Extract* works as well as steroids in reducing inflammatory responses. (See Allergic Reactions.)
- *Spilanthes Flowering Tops and Roots, Oregon Grape Root,* and *Myrrh Gum* work well together for more serious yeast and/or fungal infections.
- *Red Clover Blossoms, Stinging Nettle Leaf,* and *Cleavers* help soothe irritated tissue, often seen in severely itchy ears with rashes or tiny pimples inside and around the ear.
- *Turmeric Root, Black Catechu, Grindelia Floral Buds,* and *Lobelia* is a combination that protects the liver from circulating antigens and allergens, thereby reducing arthritic reactions as well as ear infections and skin irritations associated with a toxic response.
- *Echinacea, Red Root, Baptisia Root, Thuja Leaf,* and *Prickly Ash Bark* clean the blood and lymphatic systems, and activate the body's immune response. This combination is beneficial when the ear condition is associated with autoimmune dysfunction, which is chronic and difficult to address.
- *Sheep Sorrel, Burdock Root, Slippery Elm,* and *Turkey Rhubarb Root* is an indigenous herbal remedy for immune stimulation. Chronic cases often need this foundation for detoxification and increased resistance. Several dog breeds, such as Dalmatians, Cockers, and German Shepherds, and Siamese or Persian cats who suffer severe sensitivities or arthritis, often fail to recover until this combination is introduced. (See Immune System Dysfunction.)

Homeopathic Remedies for Ear Problems

- *Arsenicum* and *Apis* combined are effective for ear sensitivities.
- *Silica* and *Arnica* combined are effective when a hematoma (large blood blister) has formed on the ear flap.
- *Graphites* works well for foul-smelling discharge.
- *Hepar Sulph* helps sensitive, inflamed ears with discharge.
- *Rhus Tox* is indicated in chronic ear infections. It works well with *Arsenicum.*
- *Hypericum* can be used if ears are extremely sensitive to touch.

Many remedies are beneficial for both an arthritic symptom and a toxic or allergic reaction, because the underlying imbalance is the same in both cases.

Do not take ear problems lightly, as chronic inflammation and infections can lead to permanent damage, resulting in deafness. Reliance on a chemically based, medicated ear wash or drops can also permanently damage the sensitive tissues of the ear.

Ehrlichiosis (See Tick Fever.)

Emotional Problems (See Behavioral Problems.)

Eye Problems are almost always involved in curative responses and often accompany ear symptoms, since both the eyes and ears mirror liver function. Toxins can overwhelm the liver and resistance to inflammation is compromised. Check your pet's eyes daily, and wipe away any matter present. Always address eye problems quickly, as chronic irritation or infection can permanently damage the eye, possibly leading to cataract formation and even blindness.

To clean away slight discharge, use a warm, damp cotton cloth. Always use distilled water on the cloth. Wipe in the direction of the eyelashes to avoid irritating the eye further. Start in the inside corner, allow your pet to close the eye before gently wiping lightly downwards towards the outside corner.

To remove heavy matter or copious discharge, in and around the eye, use a warm, wet cotton pad or ultra-soft cotton paper towel. Hold it gently against the eye, allowing it time to soften any hardened matter. Gently wipe the inside of the lid to remove discharge on the eyeball, being careful not to introduce any dirt or crust into the eye. Then remove the remaining matter on the outside lashes. Repeat as often as needed. Do not allow the eye to remain crusted-over and shut. This will encourage infection and can damage the eye or tear duct permanently.

Follow cleaning with an application of natural eye drops made from a dilution of six drops of *Calendula Extract* in a couple of ounces of distilled water. For very irritated or dry eyes, apply a few drops of *natural Vitamin E oil*, every other day, directly to the inside of the lower eyelid. Be careful not to scratch the eye. Blinking will disperse the Vitamin E. A few drops of *Golden Seal Extract* can also be added to drops, if infection is present. This will also help to open up tear ducts, and encourage natural lubrication.

Herbal Remedies for Eye Problems

Always supplement with herbs, to strengthen and cleanse the eye, increase resistance to allergens and infections, and support anti-inflammatory and antihistamine action. Proper nutritional and herbal supplementation can prevent and even reverse cataracts, a common side effect of chronic eye irritation.

- *Yucca Extract* works as well as steroids in reducing inflammatory responses. (See Allergic Reactions.)
- *Chinese Ephedra, Mullein Leaves, and Lobelia* is a natural antihistamine combination, which quickly reduces acute responses resulting in itchy eyes and tearing. It is an excellent, short-term symptom suppressor, allowing other herbs and nutrients a chance to build up the body.
- *Eyebright, Bayberry Root, Calamus Root, Golden Seal Root*, and *Stinging Nettle Leaf* addresses symptoms that include very itchy, dry eyes, often visibly swollen, or weepy with infection.
- *Red Clover Blossoms, Stinging Nettle Leaf*, and *Cleavers* soothes irritated tissue, which can manifest as severely inflamed, itchy

eyes, with rashes or tiny pimples around the eyes, face, and ears. This herbal combination can help prevent and eliminate tiny eyelid cysts and is excellent for mange-reactive eye sensitivities.

- *Echinacea, Red Root, Baptisia Root, Thuja Leaf,* and *Blue Flag Root* clean the blood and lymphatic systems, and helps activate the body's immune response. This combination is beneficial when the eye condition may be associated with autoimmune dysfunction and can be difficult to address. Other symptoms that respond well to this combination include tiny blood blisters or cysts around the lids, often the result of trauma due to scratching.
- *Sheep Sorrel, Burdock Root, Slippery Elm,* and *Turkey Rhubarb Root* can be the key to chronic symptom reversal. (See Immune System Dysfunction.)

Homeopathic Remedies for Eye Problems

- *Arsenicum and Apis* is a great combination for sensitivities to air-borne allergens, especially itchy, runny eyes.
- *Silica and Hypericum* work together to help unblock tear ducts. Also follow directions for abscesses, if needed.
- *Euphrasia* encourages tearing to reduce dryness and irritability.
- *Pulsatilla* is indicated for creamy, profuse eye discharges.

Fatty Tumors (See Skin and Coat Problems.)

Hair Loss (See Skin and Coat Problems.)

Heart Problems, such as a rapid heartbeat, can accompany chronic arthritic reactions, which stress this organ due to powerful surges of histamine and adrenaline. Excessive panting can be mistakenly attributed to pain, yet possibly indicate a more serious heart condition, so be sure to report any changes in breathing patterns or weakness with exercise to your veterinarian.

Homeopathic Remedies for Heart Problems

If heart problems are primarily affected by pain and other arthritic reactions, then homeopathic remedies should quickly address them.

- *Aconite* is beneficial when labored breathing and tumultuous heart action follows curative response, or when heart inflammation is suspected.
- *Iberis* helps regulate an irregular heartbeat and reduce palpitations.

Hip Dysplasia (See Structural Disorders.)

Hyperparathyroidism (See Structural Disorders: Metabolic Bone Disease.)

Hypokalemia (See Structural Disorders: Metabolic Bone Disease.)

Immune System Dysfunction is often at the root of arthritic conditions. It is vital that you address and support proper immune function. Infectious arthritis can be the result of viral infections such as parvo or kennel cough, feline leukemia, or feline upper respiratory disease. Bacterial infections from tick bites can result in paralysis. Unfortunately, it is common to see pets develop more serious dis-ease, such as cancer, after struggling for years with arthritis. Many people have also reported an increase or sudden development of arthritis after the pet has been treated medically for another condition, such as kidney problems. In each case, the underlying weakness is the immune system, and the best way to reverse most symptoms is to strengthen the immune system first.

Vitamin C, A, B-Complex, and *E* cannot be surpassed for their immune-enhancing capabilities. Several other vitamins, minerals such as *Zinc*, *Selenium*, and *Chromium*, and amino acids can enhance the efficacy of these nutrients, so a properly balanced and therapeutically potent multiple supplement is essential.

In addition, several herbal and homeopathic remedies support resistance to antigens or infections, reduce catabolic waste (responsible for many arthritic symptoms), and eliminate damaged or mutated cells, which are often responsible for the development of cancerous cells and a weaken immune response.

Herbal Remedies for Immune Dysfunction

Herbal extracts, preferably organic and standardized (having a stronger, guaranteed potency), should be diluted in purified water, tuna water, or apple juice and given on an empty stomach for optimum therapeutic response. If your pet is suffering from digestive disorders, then herbs may be better tolerated when given with meals.

- *Sheep Sorrel*, *Burdock Root*, *Slippery Elm*, and *Turkey Rhubarb Root* is an old indigenous herbal remedy to eliminate catabolic waste and stimulate the immune system. Chronic cases often need this foundation for detoxification and increased resistance. Several dog breeds, such as Dalmatians, Cockers, and German Shepherds, and Siamese or Persian cats, who genetically suffer chronic immune weaknesses, which can result in arthritis, cancer, or infections, often fail to recover until this combination is introduced.

- *Echinacea* and *Golden Seal Root* are nature's antibiotics. They are effective for reversing acute symptoms of viral, bacterial, yeast, and fungal infections while stimulating the immune system in general. These natural antibiotics cleanse the blood, lymph system, liver, and kidneys. They can be used topically for the reversal of abscesses, gangrene, and pus discharge, and also to open up blocked tear ducts.

- *Astragalus Root* helps tone and stimulate the spleen, an important immune system organ. It fights infection, helps restore appetite, and reduces fatigue and diarrhea resulting from infection. It acts as a diuretic to flush wastes, reduce edema, and discharge pus, and it increases metabolism and aids the adrenals.

- *Gotu Kola* is beneficial for the whole body. It stimulates the circulation, heals nerve tissue, increases energy, is effective against over-calcification (good for hypokalemia), and combats stress. Use it both internally and topically for ringworm, hot spots, eczema, psoriasis, and staphylococcal infections. It provides excellent general support and can reverse many disabilities associated with old age.

- *Pau d'Arco* stimulates the immune system, combats infection, and relieves arthritic pain. *Pau d'Arco* is easier for very sick, weakened, or older pets to tolerate than *Golden Seal Root*. It is especially beneficial for infectious arthritis due to bacteria such as ehrlichiosis (Tick Fever).

- *Lomatium Root, Echinacea Root, Spilanthes, Chinese Schizandra Berry*, and *Licorice Root* promotes strong anti-viral activity and has immune-enhancing properties. This combination of herbs enhances cellular immunity and liver function to protect healthy cells from antigens and viral infections that trigger reactive arthritis. They are indicated in cases of chronic viral infections that have not responded well to medications, or when the liver may be inflamed—often secondary to infectious arthritis. This combination can be used with *Astragalus* for debilitating or chronic infection.

- *Echinacea, Red Root, Baptisia Root, Thuja Leaf*, and *Prickly Ash Bark* act as blood and lymphatic drainers, while activating the body's immune response. Symptoms that respond well to this combination include conditions associated with autoimmune breakdown, catabolic waste build-up, reactive arthritis, pimples/feline acne, lymphatic engorgement, chronic infection, tumor growth, cysts, fluid cysts around joints, cancer, tick fever, and wasting disease.

- *Spilanthes Leaf and Root, Grape Root, Juniper Berry, Usnea Lichen*, and *Myrrh Gum* combined are very powerful anti-fungal and anti-yeast agents. This combination is beneficial in reducing Valley Fever spore infestation that often settles in bone.

Homeopathic Remedies for Immune Dysfunction

Homeopathic remedies can facilitate the immune system's response to a specific toxin, allergen, bacterial, viral, or yeast infection, although they should never be relied upon solely to address immune imbalance. If an animal is severely debilitated, you may have no choice but to use a homeopathic remedy along with nutritional and herbal supplementation.

- *Arsenicum* quickly triggers detoxification and elimination through the liver and kidneys, and stimulates other vital organs and glands responsible for proper immune response. *Arsenicum* prepares the body to utilize immune-enhancing nutrients.

- *Gelsemium* is an outstanding remedy for the first signs of disease, especially fever. Use this remedy for pets who seem very needy and want to be held when they begin to feel poorly, or have had a relapse after a long, debilitating illness and weak recovery. Chronic infections and the early stages of Tick or Valley Fever respond well to *Gelsemium*.

- *Echinacea* is good for reoccurring infections and lymphatic engorgement. It helps address fatigue often experienced during immune problems.

- *Sweet Chestnut* is a flower remedy that addresses deep despair and anguish often experienced by a pet after a long illness.

Infections and Infectious Arthritis (See Immune System Dysfunction, Structural Disorders, Tick Fever, Valley Fever.)

Intervertebral Disc Disease (See Structural Disorders.)

Irritable Bowel Syndrome (See Colitis: IBS.)

Knees (See Structural Disorders: Cruciate Ligament.)

Lick Granuloma can develop on the body, especially around the lower legs and feet, after chronic trauma through licking has occurred. Dogs, in particular, will lick an area that might be painful or numb from arthritic disease. A hard knot slowly develops that is often the primary spot for a pet's focus. Therefore, it is commonly thought to be simply obsessive behavior, and the condition is not addressed until the granuloma appears. Once the licking has become chronic, it has also become obsessive behavior and is not addressed during treatment. Although the arthritic reaction itself has been suppressed, compulsive licking of the area will help continue the symptom cycle by re-irritating the skin. Although surgical removal of the granuloma is often the suggested course of veterinary treatment, I discourage it because it can return with a vengeance and is then more likely to become cancerous.

Licking is a serious concern for many pet owners. Excessive licking is not only irritating to the owner, it will quickly exhaust the pet. The pet's vital healing energy is redirected to address this fatigue, instead of supporting tissue repair and immune stimulation.

Although normal daily self-grooming includes licking the body clean, obsessive and chronic licking can lead to hairballs (see Digestive Disorders), skin eruptions (see Skin and Coat Problems, Allergic Reactions), even growths (see Lick Granuloma). Homeopathic *Arsenicum* works the best for constant licking, especially when a build-up of urea is involved. *St. John's Wort* and *Chamomile* help reduce the anxiety often associated with excessive licking. Try Flower Essences, such as *Rescue* or *Mimulus*, which are good for obsessive behavior. (See Allergic Reactions, Digestive Disorders.)

Liver Problems are often at the root of arthritic symptoms. The liver can become additionally burdened and congested by yeast or chemical arthritis-relief products. Eliminate all yeast at once from your pet's diet, supplements, treats, or pest control products if you suspect liver disorder.

The liver is a primary organ of the digestive, eliminatory, and immune systems. All these systems are involved in the proper functioning of the body's defenses against arthritis—especially its bone, ligament, and tissue repair capabilities. If you are to be successful in reversing your pet's arthritic condition, you will have to be truly concerned about the care and support of your pet's liver.

Herbal Remedies for Liver Problems

- *Yucca* and *Garlic Extract* are wonderful liver detoxifiers, and help reduce general inflammation and organ congestion. (See Arthritis.)
- *Lomatium Root, Echinacea Root, Spilanthes, Chinese Schizandra Berry*, and *Licorice Root* target cellular immunity and liver function to protect healthy cells from toxins. (See Immune System Dysfunction.)
- *Echinacea, Red Root, Baptisia Root, Thuja Leaf*, and *Prickly Ash Bark* act as blood and lymphatic cleansers, reducing liver toxicity. This combination reverses weakness due to hypokalemia and autoimmune reactive arthritis. (See Immune System Dysfunction.)
- *Sheep Sorrel, Burdock Root, Slippery Elm*, and *Turkey Rhubarb Root* is an old indigenous herbal remedy for catabolic waste elimination and liver stimulation. (See Digestive Disorders, Immune System Dysfunction.)

Lupus (See Immune System Dysfunction, Structural Disorders.)

Lyme's Disease (See Tick Fever.)

Masticatory Myositis (See Structural Disorders.)

Metabolic Bone Disease (See Structural Disorders.)

Mucopolysaccharidosis (See Structural Disorders.)

Muscular Problems (See Structural Disorders.)

Myositis/Myopathies (See Structural Disorders.)

Nerve Damage is a common symptom secondary to arthritis caused by calcification, muscular tension, intervertebral disc and joint disorders that impinge upon nerves. Nerve damage can result in loss of motor skills; dragging toes and stumbling is a frequent sign of nerve problems, as is poor digestion, incontinence, constipation, loss of hearing, and eventually paralysis. (See Arthritis, Paralysis, Structural Disorders.)

Obesity (See Weight Problems.)

Osteoarthritis (See Structural Disorders.)

Osteochondrosis (See Structural Disorders.)

Osteomyelitis (See Structural Disorders.)

Pancreatitis (See Digestive Disorders.)

Panosteitis (See Structural Disorders.)

Paralysis or muscular weakness can result from over-calcification (an arthritic reaction), infection (such as Tick Fever), or trauma that results in pressure on nerves. Reaction to an allergen, such as yeast, pollen, food by-products, chemicals, or medication can also create severe muscular weakness. After proper veterinarian diagnosis to rule out a viral or neurological origin, nutritional, herbal, and homeopathic remedies can reduce inflammation, pain, and debility. Often a proper course of holistic treatment can result in complete reversal of reactive paralysis.

Homeopathic *Arsenicum*, given in frequent dosages, will provide initial relief of many symptoms. *Hypericum* is indicated when nerve involvement is suspected. Taper off to two daily doses, until recovery is complete.

Yucca, in the standardized extract form only, is as effective as steroids in most applications. If needed, *Yucca* can even be used in conjunction with steroids to reduce the need for heavy doses of this potentially harmful medication, until the herb alone can be used for long-term maintenance. (See Allergic Reactions, Tick Fever.)

Patellar Luxation (See Structural Disorders.)

Potassium Depletion (See Structural Disorders: Hypokalemia.)

Rocky Mountain Spotted Fever (See Tick Fever.)

Skin and Coat Problems occur frequently with many arthritis-related conditions. The skin, the largest eliminatory organ, can manifest many symptoms due to toxicity.

Eczema, Hot Spots, Pimples, Cysts, Fatty Tumors, and *Warts* can be reversed with a combination of herbs including *Red Clover, Stinging Nettle Leaf, Cleavers Herb, Yellow Dock Root, Burdock Root*, and *Yarrow Flowers*. Homeopathically,

Apis addresses rashes and general irritation, resulting in scratching or rubbing. *Thuja* and/or *Arsenicum* help eliminate warts, cysts, and fatty growths, as does *Calcarea Carb*. *Silica* works well for eliminating growths under the skin, including cysts, abscesses, or ulcers. *Hepar Sulph* is indicated for weepy, painful areas.

Greasy Coat or Offensive Odors can be addressed through proper grooming followed by an antiseptic rinse. To make an antiseptic rinse cut up one lemon (rind and all). Boil it in one pint of distilled water for five minutes. Then cover and simmer for twenty minutes. Let the lemon sit in the water overnight. Strain in the morning and refrigerate. Add twenty drops of *Golden Seal Extract* or *Grapefruit Extract* if needed for infection control. Homeopathic *Psorinum* is beneficial when the skin has an acrid odor with discharging pustules or hot spots that are slow to heal. *Psorinum* reduces the production of the sebaceous glands, which is associated with a greasy coat and sebaceous cysts.

Dry Coat, Dandruff, Cracked Skin, and **Thin Skin** should be addressed with herbal formulas containing *Milk Thistle Seed* (for liver toxicity), *Yellow Dock Root* (improves fatty acid metabolism), *Burdock Root* (purifies blood), *Echinacea Root* (antibacterial, anti-ehrlichiosis), *Sarsaparilla Root* (for disorders associated with hormonal balance), and *Oregon Grape Root* (aids liver metabolism). *Arsenicum* is a good general homeopathic choice, while *Sepia* works well on irritations, especially cracked toes and feet, that itch badly with no relief from licking. *Psorinum* can be used for dirty and dingy coat that is brittle and lackluster. Topical application of *jojoba oil* conditioner can also help temporarily, to reduce dryness, while herbs and nutrients build-up in the body and begin to reverse the underlying imbalance.

Hair Loss, Poor Coat Condition, and ***Excessive Scratching*** respond well to *Turmeric Root, Black Catechu, Grindelia Flowers, Licorice Root, Ginkgo Leaf, African Devil's Claw, Yarrow,* and *Lobelia.* homeopathic *Arsenicum* is best suited for general hair loss. *Sulphur* addresses ringworm or other circular-patch irritations, often the cause of scratching and hair loss.

Proper grooming is of paramount importance for stimulating dead coat and skin removal and supporting circulation. Grooming will bring more nutrients to the skin and coat for tissue repair. A daily brushing followed by a rubdown with a damp terry cloth towel can work wonders. (See Allergic Reactions.)

Stomach Problems (See Digestive Disorders.)

Structural Disorders known as Osteoarthritis or degenerative joint disease describe a common condition in which the cartilage is defective or deteriorating. These conditions allow too much rotation or action in the joint capsule, resulting in bone tissue damage. Calcification occurs to repair bone, although, more commonly, over-calcification occurs resulting in stiffness, inflammation, muscular tension, and pain. *Hip Dysplasia* is a common form of degenerative joint disease. Many cases of arthritis are often due to tissue damage more than heredity. Improper nutrition, old injuries from car accidents, or physical overexertion can result in these conditions. Infectious arthritis is joint inflammation and pain due to a bacterial or viral infection.

Fever and fatigue with painfully swollen joints can accompany cases of infectious arthritis. In *Limping Kitten Syndrome*, the kitten displays generalized lameness and pain with hot, swollen joints after a bout of feline upper respiratory virus. *Polyarthritis* (affecting more than one joint) is a common reaction in pets who have been infected with various viral, bacterial, or fungal agents. Unfortunately, they may be infected by the vaccines used to prevent such diseases. (See Immune System Dysfunction, Tick Fever, Valley Fever.)

Autoimmune disease can trigger arthritic conditions. The body "attacks" itself, resulting in an abundance of antibodies bonding together within the joint, causing inflammation. The smaller breeds, such as Toy Poodles, Chihuahuas, and Min Pins are more likely to suffer autoimmune-related arthritis, while *Systemic Lupus* (another autoimmune disease) favors the larger breeds. Cat breeds, such as Abbysinian, Exotic Short Hair, and Burmese are more likely to suffer autoimmune-related arthritis, while *Systemic Lupus* seems to favor Siamese and the Oriental Short Hair. (See Cancer.)

The use of corticosteroids (anti-inflammatory drugs), and pain medication may temporarily suppress the symptoms, but do little to repair the joint or prevent further deterioration. *Glucosamine*, *Chondroitin Sulfate*, and *Manganese* combined have been well-known nutritional supplements for arthritis in holistic circles for many years. Recently, veterinarians have begun to use this "revolutionary" supplement.

Symptoms of arthritis and other structural conditions are best suppressed, and, possibly eventually reversed, homeopathically and/or herbally while the structure (joints, ligaments, muscles, and tendons) are strengthened through nutritional supplementation. (See Arthritic Reactions.) Prevention is definitely possible.

The structural or muscular conditions listed below also respond well to holistic animal care.

Cruciate ligament damage (generally a tearing or severe sprain) occurs in many pets which have not been fed the best diet nor supplemented with adequate levels of *Vitamin C* (minimum 1000 mg. per day for small pets, 2000 to 4000 mg. per day for larger dogs). Small breeds are most prone, due to their structure and also for their propensity for getting underfoot and suffering injuries. Use homeopathic *Ruta*. (See Arthritis.)

Fractures can occur due to trauma but are common in pets with nutritionally depleted and frail skeletal structures. These conditions may be due to metabolic bone disease or cancer. Symptoms include non-weight-bearing lameness, with noticeable swelling and pain. Broken bones may break through the skin or a grinding may be heard. Seek to immobilize the fractured area immediately and get to the emergency veterinary clinic. Emergency care can benefit from homeopathic support, especially *Arnica* and *Hypericum*. Follow up with increased minerals, especially *Boron* (1 to 3 mg.) and *Calcium* (250 mg. to 500 mg.) supplementation per day for the first six weeks. Utilize other supplements recommended to build stronger bones.

Hip Dysplasia is a partial dislocation of the hip joints and is genetically passed down in many popular dog breeds today including German Shepherds, Dobermans, Rottweilers, Labs, Golden Retrievers, Mastiffs, and St. Bernards. The genetic trait has become so dominant that in several breeds, particularly the Shepherds, as many as eight out of every ten pups born will develop symptoms before their second birthday! Cats can also pass this on genetically, although injury is the most common trigger for their dysplasia. Severe trauma, from a car accident, excessive exercise, or jumping can also dislocate the hips. Avoid encouraging your pet to overexert him or herself. Jumping up too high, especially straight up and down often, or excessive rotation of the limb can damage the joint and tear ligaments. Never pull your young pet by the legs, and limit exercise until they reach twelve months of age. They need this amount of time for proper growth and strengthening of the structural and muscular systems.

Most symptoms occur in pets, especially dogs, within the first six to twelve months of age. This can be due to owners who push their young pups who look grown due to their large size, but have not matured. These young tissues are sensitive to trauma. Common symptoms include walking with a great rear-end wiggle or a bunny hop and discomfort or difficulty getting up and down. If your dog is diagnosed with this condition, you must limit exercise to a few short walks per day. If the joint is pushed too far, to the point of fatigue, the tissue will begin to degenerate, resulting in inflammation and pain.

Avoid encouraging or allowing pets to run or jump about too wildly as this could trigger inflammation and pain. Swimming is an excellent way to exercise your dog while strengthening the ligaments. For the most part, cats will exercise themselves, although you should encourage movement if needed. The more you can promote strong connective tissue, the more stable the hip will remain within the joint, reducing the damage that leads to mobility difficulties, joint degeneration, calcification (from chronic bone repair) and pain.

Surgery is often sought out to stabilize the hip, but I have found that it is not as effective as holistic care in the long run, unless total dislocation has occurred. Nutritional, herbal, and homeopathic remedies provide so much more support and recovery than surgery, in a large number of severe cases.

High doses of *Vitamin C* up to bowel tolerance, or at least 2000 mg. for cats and smaller dogs to 4000 mg. for the large breeds, can help prevent hip dysplasia or at least slow down the degeneration and help relieve pain.

Legg-Perthes Disease is an orthopedic condition involving the hips that occurs in smaller breeds, such as Dachshunds, Terriers, or Miniature Poodles. It is characterized by the degeneration of the head of the femur—where the femur fits into the socket to form the hip joint. This results in general lameness and pain with standing and movement. Follow recommendations for hip dysplasia.

Intervertebral Disc Disease or *Spondylosis deformans* is a degenerative bone condition related to aging. It predominantly seems to affect large dogs, pets with long backs, or excessive jumpers. It promotes the development of bony spurs that originate from the intervertebral discs and grow to bridge the gap between adjacent vertebrae. Pain and pressure on nerves from these growths can cause prominent hind-end weakness, interfere with digestion and elimination, and can progress into paralysis if left untreated. Homeopathic treatment with *Hypericum*, *Ruta*, *Colchicum*, and *Dulcamara* is beneficial. Use *Arnica* for pain and *Yucca*, herbally, for inflammation.

Metabolic Bone Disease results in a thinning and loss of bone tissue. This leaves pets predisposed to fractures, growth deformities, and bone cancer. A common condition is *hyperparathyroidism*, is a condition in which a calcium deficiency within the bone leads to abnormal bone growth and tissue loss as the body tries to correct the calcium imbalance. This condition can be the result of a high-protein or all meat-based diet, or secondary to kidney disease, and increases the likelihood that your pet will suffer from bone cancer. A common feline condition is *mucopolysaccharidosis*, in which an enzyme deficiency leads to abnormal bone growth and tissue loss as the body tries to correct polysaccharide carbohydrate accumulation. This occurs frequently in Siamese cats (genetics). This condition increases the likelihood that your cat will suffer from bone cancer. *Boron* is a vital supplement in this condition. Herbs, including *Red Root, Thuja Leaf, Blue Flag Root*, and *Baptisia Root* are helpful in reducing bone tissue loss. *Echinacea* stimulates and balances the immune system and keeps infection from settling deeper. By slowing down the degenerative process, *Gotu Kola* benefits older pets.

Myositis triggers inflammation of the muscle tissue, resulting in stiffness, pain, weakness, and eventual muscle atrophy. Partial, short-term paralysis is not an uncommon effect of acute bouts. A feline disease, such as *hypokalemia*, which affects the heart muscles and can cause lack of coordination, difficulty eating, and weight loss, is a common side effect of potassium deficiency that can trigger overall myositis. Infectious states, including some parasitic infestations, can also trigger symptoms. These conditions are best treated individually as symptoms, rather than a disease.

Another autoimmune disease, such as *masticatory myositis* affects the facial muscles and can cause difficulty eating and drinking. It is a common hereditary trait in German Shepherds. Infectious states, including some parasitic infestations, can also trigger symptoms, which are best treated individually as symptoms, rather than a disease. Herbs, especially *St. John's Wort* and *Valerian Root*, can relax muscular stress. B-Complex and anti-oxidants also help these conditions. Massage and gentle exercise can also strengthen the muscular system and greatly improve mobility and flexibility in both these conditions.

Myopathy is the common term for generalized muscular weakness or dysfunction, and should be treated as you would myositis.

Osteochondrosis *(panosteitis: hypertrophic osteodystrophy HOD)* is a common condition characterized by abnormal growth and development of joint cartilage in young, large breed dogs, resulting in lameness and pain. Overexertion and a diet too high in protein and calories are the most common culprits. Although many parents pass this predisposition to their offspring, it can be easily prevented. Provide proper supplementation high in *Vitamin C* and *Boron*. Follow recommendations for hip dysplasia.

Osteomyelitis is the result of a deep wound, including a bite from another dog or cat, which has infected bony tissue. Open fractures also predispose a pet to infection, while fungal or bacterial organisms can spread from other parts of the body via the blood. These pets become feverish and lame, often requiring surgery to remove affected bone mass, but a holistically raised pet will, in all likelihood, be able to reverse infection prior to the onset of a serious condition. (See Immune System Dysfunction.)

Patellar Luxation is similar to hip dysplasia, but localized within the knee. Improper nutrition has left the ligaments surrounding and stabilizing the knee weakened and vulnerable to injury or degeneration. Follow recommendations for hip dysplasia.

Potassium Depletion is common in pets suffering from other diseases that result in an imbalance of vital electrolytes. Kidney or liver disease, diabetes, and cancer contribute to low potassium levels resulting in hypokalemia. Cats with Feline Infectious Peritonitis (FIP) or feline leukemia are especially prone. The long-term use of drugs to treat Feline Urological Syndrome (FUS), including urine acidifiers, has also been linked to potassium depletion. If left untreated, hypokalemia may lead to paralysis. Symptoms can include lack of coordination, muscle weakness (including in the digestive tract), constipation, loss of appetite, weight loss, and muscle pain. Intravenous injections of potassium may initially be needed, especially with the onset of respiratory paralysis, but the majority of cases respond well to oral supplementation. Since smaller pets seem to use up more potassium than the larger ones, give at least 10 mg. per day for the first week, then drop to 5 mg. per day for another week and then maintain with 3 to 5 mg. per day regardless of size. (For additional homeopathic remedies, herbs, and nutritional recommendations for bone, joint, or muscular disorders, see Arthritis.)

Tick Fever is also known as *ehrlichiosis* (most common bacteria organism), *Rocky Mountain Spotted Fever* (caused by another bacteria), or *Lyme's Disease* (the bacteria *Borrelia burgdorferi*). All are caused by a tick bite that transmits the infection. Clinical signs include anemia, loss of appetite, fever, depression, and inflammation of the joints with pain. Heavy antibiotic treatment is common although the pet often becomes worse, especially if medication is ceased. This form of infectious arthritis is easy to reverse if holistic animal care is followed. High doses of *Vitamin C* and *Garlic* supplementation in addition to specific recommendations for immune stimulation to control infection or digestive complaints, will quickly reverse a large majority of these cases completely. (See Digestive Disorders, Immune System Dysfunction.)

Ticks not only create a lot of problems related to skin problems, but also make treating arthritis impossible if infestation is allowed to continue. They weaken and infect your pet with a serious bacterial disease that can result in reactive arthritis, anemia, and ultimately paralysis. Diatomaceous earth (tiny, ground-up fossils which dehydrate the pest's outer coating and therefore kill it) can be an effective barrier between your home or yard and the pests. Clean your pet and its bedding well with a natural insecticide shampoo and follow with a natural dip. Follow all directions carefully. Groom daily to help remove pests, dead skin and coat, and also to make skin treatments easier. (See Immune System Dysfunction: Infections, Liver Problems, and Tick Fever.)

Thyroid Problems can be very common to animals that exhibit arthritic reactions, especially in addition to chronic skin conditions or weight problems. Often, thyroid problems can be caused by previous cycles of steroid medications, the drugs most commonly used to suppress arthritic symptoms.

Although it is preferable to rely on nutrients and glandulars to balance defective glands, I recommend that you consult with your veterinarian. Testing for hormonal levels will benefit you in general, regardless of what you decide to do. Utilize medication when appropriate for you and your animal, especially if nothing else seems to work.

Raw glandulars with thyroid and supportive glandulars such as adrenal and pituitary gland, plus proper nutrition, can often reverse thyroid weakness and rebalance function. *Yucca*, in the standardized extract form, seems to help the thyroid respond more quickly to nutritional support.

Herbal support includes *Bladderwrack* (for goiter, hypoactivity), and *Bugleweed*, *Motherwort*, *Lemon Balm*, *Melissa* (for hyperactivity.)

Vaccinations can trigger an arthritic reaction and weaken the immune system enough to lower resistance to toxins. If you suspect that this is the case, then use homeopathic

Arsenicum and *Thuja* in frequent daily doses until symptoms show signs of reversal. Symptoms can include lethargy, digestive upsets, including loss of appetite, and fever. You may also see a discharge from the anus, the nose, the eyes, or the injection site within twelve hours of the shots.

To use these remedies as a preventive and to lessen the likelihood of a reaction, begin dosing a few days prior to the shots. Avoid giving yearly vaccinations during the seasons your pet is most sensitive to arthritis, or avoid vaccinations altogether by researching homeopathic nosodes made from the actual diseases, such as parvo or FIP. I have had great success with this type of homeopathic protection.

Valley Fever is a serious, often-fatal, fungal infestation found in the arid southwestern states. Pets with chronic arthritic conditions are often diagnosed with Valley Fever that has settled in the bone and joints. The fungal spores (coccidioidomycosis) grow deep in dry desert dirt and are released by any type of digging. The spores are inhaled or absorbed through the skin. Treatment with chemical anti-fungal agents, such as *Nizoral*, often suppresses symptoms only to have them return with a vengeance once medication is ceased.

The side effects of anti-fungal drugs can be permanently damaging to the liver and kidneys, as well as causing suppression of the immune system. Therefore, it is not uncommon for these pets to suffer reactive paralysis, or, at the very least, have an aggravation of chronic arthritic symptoms.

Veterinarian diagnosis and follow-up through blood work is important, as is a strict holistic lifestyle.

Herbal treatment is effective in reversing the fungal count. Often, the count may end up in the low end, 1:4, but it will never reach zero since the body retains antibodies. Nevertheless, a holistically supported pet can remain free of symptoms or weakness, regardless of this "positive" titer count.

Herbal Remedies for Valley Fever

- *Garlic Extract* has anti-fungal activity and is very valuable to use for Valley Fever and related symptoms, including lack of appetite or other digestive disorders.
- *Yucca Extract* relieves the inflammatory response often associated with Valley Fever, since the spore infestation can settle within the brain, lungs, bones, and joints.
- *Spilanthes Leaf and Root, Grape Root, Juniper Berry, Usnea Lichen*, and *Myrrh Gum*, combined, are very powerful anti-fungal and anti-yeast agents, and are beneficial in reducing Valley Fever spore infestation and secondary infections. (See Immune System Dysfunction.)

Vomiting (See Digestive Disorders.)

Weight Problems are not uncommon in pets who also have arthritic symptoms. Improper digestion and assimilation (also at the root of arthritis) can interfere with the body's ability to utilize calories properly for energy. The brain is responsible for deciding if the body is being fed enough. If nutrients are not available to the blood through proper assimilation, the brain will think that the body is starving and decide to store calories as fat, rather than use them as energy to repair tissue and support the immune system. Pets who suffer great pain, anxiety, or debilitation along with their structural disorders, can also have trouble maintaining proper weight, regardless of what they are fed.

Allowing your pet to remain overweight will only serve to make the arthritis worse. Stress on the structure, especially joint supporting ligaments, is constant and can cause degeneration of the structural support system. Torn ligaments, stiff joints, and the loss of mobility will only increase your pet's discomfort and interfere with its curative potential.

Herbs, such as *Chickweed, Safflower Flowers, Burdock Root, Parsley, Licorice Root, Hawthorne Berries, Fennel,* and *Cayenne* work together to melt pounds away naturally and rebalance the digestive tract for greater assimilation.

Siberian Ginseng, Chinese Schizandra Berry, Damiana Leaf, Kola Nut, Wild Oats, Skullcap, and *Prickly Ash* work synergistically to restore integrity to the adrenal glands and promote weight gain and maintenance. This herbal combination acts as an adaptogen to counter chronic stress or pain, which may be causing weight loss due to arthritic reactions. (See Digestive Disorders.)

Wobbler's Syndrome is caused by vertebral instability, resulting in nerve damage, lack of coordination, and hind-end paralysis. Several breeds, particularly Doberman Pinschers, Great Danes, and German Shepherds, are genetically prone to this disorder but others may develop it after trauma to the neck. Choke chain collars and rough handling of puppies in training can predispose dogs to this disorder. Although severe cases may warrant surgery to relieve spinal cord pressure, holistic animal care has successfully reversed or slowed the degenerative effects of this disorder. (See Nerve Damage.)

How to Be Your Vet's Best Friend

The most important ally that you can have, in taking care of your pet, is a trusted veterinarian. You should never think that you can handle each and every health concern on your own. You can however, manage your pet's health care yourself, while making all medically-related decisions using the expertise and guidance of a competent professional. Rely on your veterinarian to explain specific genetic weaknesses and local health concerns so that you can develop a sound preventative program around your pet's individual needs.

Yearly health exams and occasional blood work can help catch an imbalance early, before it becomes a health problem. Often an imbalance in the endocrine system, protein assimilation, or blood sugar irregularities can be spotted long before the actual symptoms, such as allergies or organ failure, show themselves. This can make the difference between simply reversing an acute weakness or having a chronic condition develop. Proper diagnosis to verify a specific imbalance can make the difference between addressing the problem head-on and more successfully, or trying a "hit or miss" therapy that can go on for months. Monitoring the body as it responds to the chosen therapy will also help you identify generally what is or isn't working.

Today, there are more holistically-oriented veterinarians who are well versed in the complementary modalities of nutritional therapy, herbs, homeopathy, acupuncture, massage and chiropractic care. Some have even expanded to incorporate esoteric therapies of sound, light and energy healing. In addition, a large number of allopathic (traditionally trained) veterinarians now realize that natural pet care has its place within their traditional, medically-based treatments.

Unfortunately, many of us have had very negative experiences with veterinarians—especially those allopathically trained veterinarians who are unfamiliar with natural care and thus are uncompromising. We may now avoid seeking veterinary support. Possibly, they have spoken to us as if we did not have a clue in our heads about our pet's health care needs, or dismissed our attempts to seek a chemical-free lifestyle for our pets. More likely, they simply failed to address past conditions successfully, and we have lost faith in the medical approach. I am hoping that by giving you a little insight as to what can be successfully accomplished with natural modalities, while encouraging you to join forces with your veterinarian—rather than give them unchallenged authority over your pet's medical care—will help empower you so that you can successfully incorporate proper veterinary care in your pet's holistic lifestyle.

It is vital that you seek a veterinarian who is willing to listen to you, is thorough in their examination and diagnosis, will explain what it is that they recommend and why—but most importantly—will treat you and your pet with respect. If you do not like the way a veterinarian approaches your pet or speaks to you, then find another no matter who recommended them.

It becomes very frustrating for a diagnostician when a pet owner doesn't have the most basic information, and puts the veterinarian (who cares) at a disadvantage—in properly identifying what might be a the bottom of the pet's symptoms. Soon, such veterinarians become jaded and assume that all their clients simply don't have a clue. Who can blame them? Open the lines of communication. Learn more about the choices you make and the recommendations given to you by all concerned parties. You know your pet best and this information will help your companion receive better veterinary care.

By making the necessary changes in their lifestyle and health care before a serious problem or chronic condition develops, you will keep them healthy. Prevention is the best cure!

The best defense for an arthritic pet is a strong offense. The first step is to get a proper diagnosis from your veterinarian to ensure that you are not dealing with a more serious illness or structural disorder. Whatever the problem, serious or minor, there are many natural protocols you and your veterinarian can successfully follow.

Above all, do not give up prematurely. There are no magic bullets. Remember that the more compromised an animal's health is and the longer they have been suffering, the longer it will take to rebalance the body—but nature holds the key.

THE CROSSING PRESS POCKET PET SERIES

Allergies
By Lisa Newman
$6.95 • Paper • ISBN 1-58091-002-5

Natural Dog
By Lisa Newman
$6.95 • Paper • ISBN 1-58091-000-9

Natural Cat
By Lisa Newman
$6.95 • Paper • ISBN 1-58091-001-7

Nutrition
By Lisa Newman
$6.95 • Paper • ISBN 1-58091-004-1

Parasites
By Lisa Newman
$6.95 • Paper • ISBN 1-58091-006-8

Skin & Coat Care
By Lisa Newman
$6.95 • Paper • ISBN 1-58091-008-4

Training without Trauma
By Lisa Newman
$6.95 • Paper • ISBN 1-58091-007-6

OTHER CROSSING PRESS PET BOOKS

Psycho Kitty?
Understanding Your Cat's Crazy Behavior
By Pam Johnson-Bennett

Is your cat's behavior making you crazy? Johnson-Bennett believes that trying to understand how your cat thinks is a key to your cat's misbehavior. She shares real cases to illustrate various problems and explains how she arrives at an appropriate solution through behavior modification.

$12.95 • Paper • ISBN 0-89594-909-1

Twisted Whiskers
Solving Your Cat's Behavior Problems
By Pam Johnson

Johnson's cat-friendly, no-nonsense techniques glow with common sense and insight…a practical guide and an inspiration.

$12.95 • Paper • ISBN 0-89594-710-2

To receive a current catalog from The Crossing Press
please call toll-free, 800-777-1048.
www.crossingpress.com

7 42851 00695 3   00033>